Advice to the Healer

Richard Colgan

Advice to the Healer

On the Art of Caring

Second Edition

 Springer

Richard Colgan
University of Maryland
Baltimore, MD, USA

ISBN 978-1-4614-5169-3   ISBN 978-1-4614-5170-9 (eBook)
DOI 10.1007/978-1-4614-5170-9
Springer New York Heidelberg Dordrecht London

Library of Congress Control Number: 2012945593

Printed on acid-free paper

Springer is part of Springer Science+Business Media (www.springer.com)

This book is dedicated to the most important teachers in my life: my wife Deborah Ann, my children Kathleen, Michael, and Conor; Eileen Rooney and my parents John J. and Anna P. Colgan. I will be eternally grateful for their love

Preface

I am grateful for the success of "Advice to the Young Physician: On the Art of Medicine." This has given me the opportunity to write a second edition. I reviewed the first edition and recognized that most of the material was applicable not just to young physicians but physicians and clinicians of all ages. There was also a need to broaden the diversity of figures highlighted. Therefore, the second edition has been substantially augmented with material that looks to reach a wider audience. Clinicians have a lot in common. We can and do learn from each other. Physicians, nurses, dentists, pharmacists, social workers, psychologists, physician assistants, nurse practitioners, and others are collectively joined in a unique brother and sisterhood. They have responded to a calling to care for our fellow men and women. This second edition was written to inspire all clinicians, young and not so young.

One reviewer noted that the first edition was really two small books in one. He was right. To highlight this duality, the second edition has been divided into two sections. Part I focuses on inspirational perspectives from history to include new healers. In Part II, I have expanded on inspirational advice for the modern-day healer.

A major change in the second edition is the inclusion of material that highlights women and healers from other cultures and caring professions. Here are some brief descriptions of this new material:

- There were no women highlighted in the first book. In researching the women who have been most influential to us in the caring profession, one woman stood out from the rest—Florence

Nightingale. Because clinicians have much to learn from "the woman with the lamp," I have included a chapter about her fascinating life.

- The intriguing and inspirational stories of "The Three Physicians of Jian An" were added, highlighting the benefits we enjoy to this day from the contributions of ancient Chinese medicine.
- Although we are not therapists we do counsel, and therefore I have added a section on the clinician as counselor.
- The section on Osler has been expanded to include many of the keen observations made by Charles S Bryan.
- Osler also noted that it was Imhotep who "was the first physician to stand out in the midst of antiquity," and I think you will enjoy the chapter on the everlasting contributions which this Egyptian physician made to the field of medicine.

So much of what is communicated in the consultation room or on the wards of a hospital between a patient and his or her physician, nurse, or therapist is the telling of a story. Our ability to appreciate these stories helps not only the patient but enriches us immeasurably. I have added two stories of patients which I think will entertain and educate you. You'll read about a special love between Joe and Elsie in "A Modern Family" and what keeps Ted, a man suffering from tardive dyskinesia, alive in "A Meaningful Life."

Few things stop and give me reason to pause more than when I hear about the incredible acts of kindness and caring by ordinary practitioners. I wanted to highlight the extraordinary random acts of kindness and the daily practices of unselfishness and altruism shown by non-famous clinicians. In "Unsung Heroes and Heroines," you will read about the greatness of those who are anonymous but to their own patients. In addition to the original material included in the first edition, I've also included an image of the painting "The Doctor" by Sir Luke Fildes. The reader will feel like he or she is standing in the dirt floor cottage with this healer as I review the iconography of what has been one of the most influential works of art showcasing the field of medicine.

Baltimore, MD, USA   Richard Colgan

Acknowledgments
for the First Edition

It would be impossible to write a book that involves so many great historical figures without the expertise of others with more knowledge in those respective areas. Foremost, I thank my colleague Milford Foxwell for gifting me with Francis Adam's translation of *The Genuine Works of Hippocrates* and *Peabody's Doctor and Patient*, as well as sharing his excitement of the history of medicine with me. I am equally grateful to another University of Maryland School of Medicine faculty member, Dr. Philip Mackowiak, for his insights and personal recollections of Dr. Theodore Woodward. I would like to acknowledge my mentors, as a student and as a young physician, Dr. Joseph Lombard and Mary Lombard, Drs. David Schneiderman, Michael Berard, and Melvin Sharoky as well as C. Earl Hill. I thank my teachers in private practice Drs. Michael J. LaPenta, William A. Dabbs, R. Scott Eden, Elizabeth Fronc, and Lisa Murray. I am indebted to my current role models at the University of Maryland School of Medicine, including Vice President for Medical Affairs and Dean E. Albert Reece, our Departmental Chairman David L. Stewart, and the entire faculty of the Department of Family and Community Medicine. I am particularly grateful to the medical students and residents of the University of Maryland School of Medicine who have taught and continue to teach me—one of whom was David Edwards who suggested undertaking this project. I thank Pamela Miller, from the Osler History of Medicine Library at McGill University, for her assistance in researching the life of Sir William Osler and for providing me with archival photos. Lachlan Forrow,

President of The Albert Schweitzer Fellowship, was gracious in both assisting me with information about Albert Schweitzer and allowing me access to photos. My appreciation to Zoe Agoos, from Partners In Health, Boston, MA, for her guidance in helping me learn more about Dr. Paul Farmer and his organization. Gregory Makoul, Chief Academic Officer at Saint Francis Hospital and Medical Center, was kind enough to allow me to include some of his important work on communication skills. I appreciate the counsel and attention to details given to me by Senior Editor Laura Walsh and Editorial Assistant Maureen Tobin from Springer Publishers. Robert B. Taylor and Richard G. Roberts have been extremely generous with their time in providing feedback and offering direction on this manuscript. Imperfections which remain are my responsibility and not theirs. My thanks go to Daniel and Gerard Ricciotti for their expert Web designing and videography support. I am especially grateful to the careful review, editing, and suggestions offered by Caitlin Iafolla Zaner—a young healer—whose expertise greatly improved the quality of the book you are about to read.

Lastly but in no way least, I want to acknowledge the most important teachers in my life: John J. and Anna P. Colgan. Together with Eileen Rooney, my wife Deborah, our children Kathleen, Michael, and Conor, along with my brother John and sisters Jadean, Patricia, and Regina I have learned what love means.

Acknowledgements
for the Second Edition

Dr. Lixing Lao is a senior researcher with The Center for Integrative Medicine and directs the center's research program in Traditional Chinese Medicine at the University of Maryland School of Medicine. He and Dr. Marta Hanson, Professor of History of Medicine at Johns Hopkins University, provided helpful insights into the contributions of traditional Chinese medicine. My wife, Deborah Colgan, a home health nurse and loving human being, cowrote the chapter on Florence Nightingale with me. I thank Dr. Charles S. Bryan for his interest in Osler and mentorship. His book *Osler: Inspirations from a Great Physician* was a great resource in enabling me to expand this chapter. Dr. Adrienne Williams, Director of Behavioral Science in the Department of Family and Community Medicine at the University of Maryland School of Medicine, was kind enough to provide very helpful edits to the chapter on Clinician as Counselor. Last but in no way least, I appreciate the guidance which Springer Editor Katharine Cacace and Developmental Editor Mary Meritt have given me.

Contents

Part I   Inspirational Perspectives from History

1   Introduction...   3
   References...   9
   Further Reading and Resources   10

2   Ancient Times...   11
   Imhotep (2655–2600 BC)   11
   Hammurabi   13
   Hippocrates   15
      The Hippocratic Oath...   20
   Early Greeks..   24
   References...   27
   Imhotep   28
   Hammurabi   28
   Siddartha   28
   Hippocrates   28
   Early Greeks..   29
   History of Medicine   29

3   Chinese and Medieval Medicine   31
   Three Divine Doctors of Jian An   31
      Zhang Zhongjing...   31
      Hua Tuo..   32
      Dong Feng..   33

Rhazes 34

Avicenna.. 37

Maimonides.. 39

The Physician's Oath and Prayer of Maimonides.............. 41

    The Oath of Maimonides 41

    The Prayer of Maimonides... 42

References.. 44

Three Divine Physicians of Jian An................................. 44

Rhazes 44

Avicenna.. 45

Maimonides.. 45

4   The Twentieth Century.. 47

Florence Nightingale.. 47

Florence Nightingale's Notes on Nursing

Which Apply to the Art of Caring 50

Santa Filomena.. 52

Sir William Osler 53

    Manage Time Well: Day-Tight Compartment 60

    Find a Calling: Being True to Certain Ideals 62

    Find Mentors: The Young Person's Friend 63

    Be Positive: "Prince of Friends and Benefactors" 64

    Learn and Teach: Drive Plato's Horses.......................... 65

    Care Carefully: The Least Sentimental

    and the Most Helpful 65

Francis Weld Peabody... 67

Albert Schweitzer.. 70

References.. 75

Nightingale... 76

Osler.. 76

Ask Osleriana—A Searchable Database

of Osler Essays.. 77

Schweitzer.. 77

The Albert Schweitzer Institute 78

5   Modern Masters... 79

Theodore E. Woodward 79

Edmund D. Pellegrino... 82

Principles of Medical Ethics 89

Paul Farmer 91

Unsung Heroes and Heroines.. 96
    The Primacy of the Trusted Healing Relationship......... 97
The Gift of Time 99
Elasticity 100
Access 101
Care for the Patient 101
References... 102
Further Reading and Resources 103
Resource... 103

Part II   Practical Advice for the Modern-Day Healer

6   **Survival Tips for the Younger Clinician** 107
    The Art of Presentation.. 107
    Practice Makes for Better Practice.................................... 113
    Good Communication... 116
    The Kalamazoo Consensus Statement............................... 117
        Essential Elements of Communication
        in Medical Encounters 117
    References... 118
    How to Present 119
    Practice Makes for Better Practice.................................... 119

7   **Civility**.. 121
    The Six Habits of Highly Respectful Physicians.............. 122
    The 25 Rules of Considerate Conduct Abridged
    for the Healer 123
    References... 129
    Civility 129

8   **Lessons Learned from Private Practice** 131
    The Clinician as Counselor.. 131
    How to BATHE Your Patients as You SOAP Them 134
    Choosing Good Practice 135
    Definition of Malpractice... 135
    Common Lawsuits 136
    Missed Myocardial Ischemia 136
    Missed Acute Abdomen.. 137
    Failing to Inform Your Patients That
    They Are at High Risk 137

What Your Defense Attorney Wants You to Know............ 138
References.. 140
Clinicians as Counselors... 141

9   **A Doctor's Journal**.. 143
Searching for the True Poetry of Life 143
Recollections.. 144
Poems from Private Practice 146
He Apologized, Twice.. 147
A Modern Family... 150
A Meaningful Life 154
References.. 158
Searching for the True Poetry of Life 158
A Meaningful Life 158
A Doctor's Journal 159

10 **Heal Thyself**.. 161
Reference 164
Further Reading and Resource... 164

11 **The Healer** 165
The Healer as a Person... 168
The Healer–Patient Interaction 168
The Healer's Vocation.. 169
The Doctor—Sir Luke Fildes... 171
A Healer's Prayer... 173
References.. 174
Further Reading and Resources 174

Index.. 175

Part I
Inspirational Perspectives from History

Chapter 1
Introduction

He knew his art, but not his trade

–Jonathan Swift

John Arbuthnot (1667–1735) was a writer who also served as physician to Queen Anne of England at the turn of the eighteenth century. Recognized by his friends, the English poet Alexander Pope and Anglo-Irish satirist Jonathan Swift, to possess great wit and compassion, John Arbuthnot was not always conscientious about his business affairs and as a writer he often allowed others to take credit for his work. [1] Swift noted that Arbuthnot was "singularly careless of his literary fame, published his best things anonymously, and let his friends edit and alter them at will." [1] Upon the death of Queen Anne, Arbuthnot and other members of the queen's court were discharged. Swift lamented this change for Arbuthnot was known for practicing the art of medicine and proclaimed "He knew his art but not his trade." [1] Evidently, the distinguished court physician was not an impressive businessman; this aspect of his profession suffered as he focused solely on the care of his patients. Nevertheless, his nurturing and benevolent characteristics were recognized by his patients and society alike. These values persist to modern day, for it is understood that one of the highest accolades a patient can give his physician is that he or she practices the *art* of medicine.

R. Colgan, *Advice to the Healer: On the Art of Caring*,
DOI 10.1007/978-1-4614-5170-9_1,
© Springer Science+Business Media, LLC 2013

I have practiced medicine for 25 years and have taught for most of
that time. Still, I know that I have not fully mastered the *art* of medicine. However, I think I know something about you, the reader. Each
of you knows the importance of mastering the art and is aware of its
critical role in delivering humanistic patient-centered care. Yet I suspect you recognize that there is much more to learn. You may view
yourself as an incomplete physician or clinician from another clinical
background. You are idealistic and strive to be a "good doctor," and
you truly care about caring for others.

We come from differing fields: medicine, nursing, dentistry, pharmacy, social work, clinical psychology, optometry, and podiatry, to
name a few. What we have in common is that we care and do so by
providing clinical care. Like those in teaching and law, we are members of the learned professions and, of course, deserve our distinct
recognitions earned through years of hard work and rigorous education. For the purposes of this book, I am going to simplify matters by
referring to the readers as a collective *healer*, since this is the princi-
pal group for which I have written. The subject matter in the chapters
to follow focuses at times on medicine, nursing, or psychology but
applies to the wealth of interdisciplinary occupations known as the
healing professions. In the pages to follow you'll read advice and
recommendations made by physicians to physicians and other greats
in different health care specialties to members of their healing professions. A premise of this second edition is that we in the healing professions have much to learn from each other. We are all incomplete
healers.

You likely chose medicine, nursing, social work, or another caring
profession as a career for many reasons, including a love for science,
a respect for mathematics, and an interest in helping others. Maybe
you are a natural-born surgeon who always loved tinkering, building
things, and solving problems. One of the premises of this book is that
the best healers, at least the ones who I would want to be associated
with, are lovers of the humanities, of humankind, of *people*. Yet
somewhere along the way in your education you have surely noticed
a large emphasis on the science — numbers, tests, studies, metrics —
and find yourself wanting more of the human side of medicine, the
people side. You long to learn more about *the art of caring*.

I want to tell you how I gained interest in this subject. Between
college and medical school, I dabbled in the study of science and
considered dedicating my life to this very technical, concrete field.

In my interview for a PhD position in Biochemistry at the University of Florida, the chairman said to me, "You look like a people person." I beamed and proudly said, "Yes, I am." He then said, 'We are not looking for "people persons' here. We're looking for someone we can put in a lab and several months later he'll come out with the answer." I was rejected as an applicant to the University of Florida, only to be accepted into a PhD program in Biochemistry at Johns Hopkins University. Six months later I left Hopkins, for I was indeed a people person and felt stifled by the confinements of the lab. This book is meant for those who recognize themselves as people persons, for those who see value in the delivery of humanistic health care, and for those who want to hone the skills necessary to practice the art of caring, be it in medicine or another one of the healing professions.

After residency I joined a group of three established physicians, particularly because I wanted to learn from those with greater experience in the practice of medicine. I considered myself well adapted to the intellectual and emotional demands of being a physician, yet I did not appreciate how much I had to learn until the respected senior partner told me upon joining the practice, "Don't be discouraged, in about 10 years you'll get in your groove!" Ten years later, I knew he was right. In order to become a better physician, the practice of medicine takes extensive and diligent training, life-long learning, and dedication to the pursuit of evidence-based medicine, as taught by colleagues, students, and patients. After 12 years in private practice, I was given the opportunity to return to academia and pursue a long-standing dream of teaching. I am now in a position to be able to observe firsthand much of what students and residents are taught.

In order to expose third-year medical students to many of the ideas presented in this book, I developed a workshop in our primary care clerkship that focuses on establishing and nurturing the physician–patient relationship. For many years, I considered assembling these ideas into a book and was compelled to do so after an MD/PhD student approached me at the end of our clerkship. After expressing similar appreciations he said, "You should write a book, Dr. Colgan." He told me that most young researchers are aware of a book by Santiago Ramon y Cajal entitled *Advice for a Young Investigator*, and there was not yet a similar book for physicians or medical students. I was amazed to find this to be the case. I believe that the points made in this book are important for all healers, and therefore I committed myself to taking on this task.

Professor Henry Hartshorne taught his medical students at the Women's Medical College of Pennsylvania in 1872, "Medicine is indeed a science but its practice is an art."[2] The science behind the healing arts is clearly important but not the focus of this book. Rather we will pursue the concept of the *art of caring,* much of which is not within the scientific realm. I am referring to the interactions between clinician and patient, that which falls under the umbrella of humanism. It embodies the stylistic ways in which kindhearted and open-minded clinicians practice these traits and signifies the mastery of skill needed for its successful application. Furthermore, this concept entails the more abstract tips, pearls, anecdotes, aphorisms, and best-practiced lessons from exceptional and experienced clinicians—those which rarely get disseminated in a formal way to today's healers and healers in training. Understanding the art of caring raises thought to multiple questions. How it is that someone can meet a physician (or nurse, social worker, psychologist, etc.) and within a few moments conclude that he or she is a good clinician? What happens during an exam room consultation that makes one patient want to follow the clinician's advice and another go running for the door? How do we connect with our patients? Why do we want to connect with our patients, and—most importantly—how can we do these things better?

The American educator Francis Weld Peabody communicated "the essential quality of a physician is an interest in humanity."[3] Perhaps the single greatest question this book will address is: How can we better show our patients our concern for their humanity? Likewise, how can clinicians accomplish this while helping others gain freedom from disease and attain their best possible health? I propose the foundation to this answer is indeed the science behind each of our respective fields. Knowledge learned from completion of thousands of clinical trials and randomized studies and the intricate scope explored through such technological advancements as electron microscopy and the molecular analysis of the human genome are examples of the *science* of medicine, which has advanced our health. Of course, these must be recognized for their contribution to effective medical practice. My goal is to convey that there is more to medicine than the science, and this notion stems from thousands of years of clinical practice and teaching. Even the best practitioners of pure science are incomplete physicians. To be complete physicians we must appreciate and excel in the art of medicine. To be complete healers we must appreciate and excel in the art of caring. We must learn how to best use this science for each patient and for humankind as a whole, through effective communication, respect, and understanding. Not only this, but we must recognize that the technologies available to restore the health of patients are applied not only to disease processes or organ systems, but to people—with unique backgrounds, cultural values, educations, and life experiences.

Throughout medical school, residency, specialties, and subspecialties some feel we have allowed the science to overshadow the art. Understandably, the art of medicine is not formally taught to the young physician or physician-in-training. At a minimum, this abstract notion is relegated to passing comments from senior to junior physicians. An example of what such a dialogue might sound like follows:

> Junior physician: "How did you get such good judgment?"
> Senior physician: "Good experience."
> (Long pause)
> Junior physician: "How did you gain such good experience?"
> Senior physician: "Bad judgment."

This is an example of one of the many ways that junior physicians (medical students, residents, fellows, and those beginning practice) learn the art of medicine—a side comment in the hall, an informal conversation, the dispensing of a clinical pearl here and there. The main reason why I chose to write this book is because this style of learning—while incredibly valuable—is not universal or consistent, nor are the same critically important lessons taught to each student clinician. Some academic medical educators might rightfully argue that such a broad ambition, with a goal of improving outcomes, should not be undertaken unless you have metrics, proven pilot studies, or other data to show that this manner of medical education is "validated." I do not have these things, and I respectfully continue with my goals. Thus, the disclaimer of this book might begin with the fact that this text may not stand up to the rigors of proper pedagogical good form. I acknowledge this, yet I prefer to view the lack of empirical evidence for this form of teaching as testimony to my point that we need to generate a greater discussion of these subjects in medical education. I maintain that we must start somewhere—somehow—to fill in this gap. I aim to introduce you to what I believe are some of the most important teachings on the physician–patient relationship as they exist throughout medical history.

Medical schools across the country are evolving to include more on the art of medicine in their curricula. They accomplish this with varying courses such as "Introduction to Clinical Medicine," "The Physician and Patient in Society," and "Doctor and Patient". These efforts are excellent, are admirable, and vary from school to school. Extracurricular efforts, as exemplified by the impressive growth of the Gold Humanism Honor Society, for example, and other professionalism efforts are to be lauded as well. They are a start, an important start, but, like us, they are incomplete.

So why read this book? First, I believe that all physicians and other clinicians want to be the best they can be. To be a great physician — a true healer — you must be mindful of the tremendous impact which the art of medicine has on the entirety of medical practice. Second, it has been my experience that, generally speaking, most physicians are only vaguely familiar with many of the most important lessons from the greatest teachers of medicine. Third, I believe there exists among physicians a common recognition of insufficiency in their education about the art of medicine; moreover, this unfortunate acknowledgement ignites their aspiration for further learning. We have so much to learn from those who came before us. This is what I aspire to teach you.

We will trace some of the most basic of caring methods back to ancient Egypt. We will explore what Hippocrates, the Father of Medicine, had to say beyond "*First do no harm*."[4] We will answer many questions along the way. What did the Greeks and others of Aristotle's time have to teach us about the art of medicine? We will explore traditional Chinese medicine to see what they have contributed to conventional medicine as well as public health. We will learn how Florence Nightingale cared for her soldiers one at a time while also being a tremendous influence on the nascent discipline of public health and biostatistics. Why is it that you cannot do a rotation in internal medicine without hearing the Canadian medical educator Sir William Osler's name mentioned at least once? Who was he and what was he trying to teach us about being a complete physician? I will introduce you to other greats, such as the previously mentioned American educator Francis Weld Peabody, who had much more to say beyond his most famous quote, "The secret in the care of the patient is to care for the patient." [3] We will explore recurring themes of which some of the greatest educators spoke, such as the value of listening to the patient, the demands and rewards of being in the service industry, and why after all is said and done everything we do must come down to taking care of one very important person: our patient. The American writer and physician Daniel Watts reminds us of what literature can do for medicine by referencing Tolstoy's three questions: [5]

> What is the most important time?
> Now, no other time matters.
> Who is the most important person?
> The one you are with.
> What is the most important thing to do?
> To do good for that person.

I recognize that this book is but one physician's viewpoint of the art of caring, as exemplified by some of the greatest healers and educators known to mankind. The list is incomplete and qualitative, not quantitative.

I share with you what I believe to be compilations of some of the greatest medical teachers, those who I consider to have exceptional words of wisdom to pass along to all of us. I have much to learn. So do you. But that should not stop us. In the words of English poet and playwright Robert Browning (1812–1889), as he wrote of the poet and scholar Abraham ibn Esra (1092–1167) in the poem *Rabbi Ben Ezra*, I confess to you, "That which I have strived to be, and am not, comforts me." [6] We have an ethical duty to our patients and society to strive for greatness in our professional practice. We must attempt to achieve the lessons of French sculptor Rodin who reminds us, "Love your calling with a passion. It is the meaning of your life." [7] Perhaps after reading this book your colleagues and patients will notice a difference in the way you practice your vocation, commit to your patient, and strive to connect on a human level in order to provide the best possible care. Above all, my wish for you is that your patients will describe you as someone who "knew the art, but not his (or her) trade." [1]

References

1. Patrick D. Chambers cyclopedia of English literature. Philadelphia, PA/London: J.B. Lippincott Company/W & R Chambers Limited; 1902. p. 145.
2. Hartshorene H. Valedictory address, 1872 sympathy and science women physicians in American medicine. New York: Oxford University Press; 1985.

3. Peabody FW. Doctor and patient. New York: The Macmillan Company; 1930.
4. Adams F. The genuine works of hippocrates. New York: Krieger Pub Co; 1972.
5. Watts D. What literature can do for medicine: a starting point. In: The examined life, vol 1, Number 3. Iowa: The University of Iowa Carver College of Medicine in Iowa City; 2012. http://theexaminedlifejournal.blogspot.com
6. Browning R. Rabbi Ben Ezra. In: Nicholson DHS, Lee AHS, editors. The oxford book of English mystical verse. Oxford: The Clarendon Press; 1917.
7. Rodin A. Providence Express. 2009. http://www.express.org.au/article.aspx?aeid=3246. Accessed May 2009

Further Reading and Resources

8. Hahn FW. The art of medicine. Kansas City: Leathers Publishing; 2006.
9. Lacombe M. On being a doctor. Philadelphia, PA: American College of Physicians; 1995.
10. Lown B. The lost art of healing: practicing compassion in medicine. New York: Ballantine Books; 1999.
11. Lyons AS. Medicine: an illustrated history. New York: Harry N. Abrams Inc; 1978.
12. Ratzan RM, Carmichael A. Medicine, a treasury of art and literature. New York: Harkavy Publishing Service; 1991.
13. Ramon y Cajal S. Advice for a young investigator. Cambridge: MIT Press; 2004. Trans. N. Swanson and L. Swanson.
14. Reynolds R, Stone J. On doctoring. New York: Simon & Schuster; 2001.
15. Wear D, Bickel J. Educating for professionalism: creating a culture of humanism in medical education. Iowa: University of Iowa Press; 2008.
16. Books A. The art and science of being a doctor: leading doctors reveal the secrets to professional and personal success as a doctor. Boston, MA: Aspatore Books; 2002.
17. Cassell EJ. The healers art. Cambridge, MA: The MIT Press; 1985.

Chapter 2
Ancient Times

Imhotep (2655–2600 BC)

The first figure of a physician to stand out clearly from the mists of antiquity.

— Sir William Osler

We must look at many historical figures in order to best understand what it means to be a healer and how to best practice the art of caring. Sir William Osler recommended that we "must come to the land of the Nile for the origin of many of man's most distinctive and highly cherished beliefs" [1]. Osler urges us to pay attention to the contributions of Imhotep—and I am.

Imhotep, who lived in the twenty-seventh century BC, was an Egyptian polymath considered to be the first architect, engineer, and physician in recorded history. He was also revered as a philosopher and one of only a few commoners ever to be acknowledged by the Egyptian people as having divine status after his death. Imhotep was also deified by the Greeks as Asclepius, the god of healing.

Imhotep stood out from the mists of antiquity in part because his practices were unlike others of his era. They were devoid of magical thinking. The Egyptians of his time thought that most illnesses (aside from trauma) were expressions of hostility by a higher power, e.g., an adversary, a spirit, or a dead person. The Ebers Papyrus, not felt to be authored by Imhotep but reflective of the type of medicine practiced in ancient Egypt, contained primarily magical remedies to help with suffering. An Egyptian might have sought out a magician or a priest

R. Colgan, *Advice to the Healer: On the Art of Caring*,
DOI 10.1007/978-1-4614-5170-9_2,
© Springer Science+Business Media, LLC 2013

as readily as a physician for a cure. "The border between magic and medicine is a modern invention; such distinction did not exist for ancient healers," noted Dr. Axel Karenberg, a medical historian, and Dr. C. Leitz, an Egyptologist, both of the University of Cologne, Germany [2].

According to Egyptologist Bob Biers in his book *Ancient Egyptian Magic*, "Some evidence exists that the kind of illness determined the method of treatment. If the cause was known, as in the case of broken bones and such perils as crocodile bites, then the treatment tended to be nonmagical. For instance, for a crocodile bite, a practical suggestion was to sew the wound closed and place raw meat on it. If, however, the illness was something such as a fever, where the cause would be unknown to the Egyptians, then it might be attributed to demons or malicious magic" [3].

There are no known writings of Imhotep, but The Edwin Smith Surgical Papyrus, one of the most important documents describing medicine in the ancient Nile Valley, has been attributed to him. The Smith Papyrus was written around 1700 BC and describes wounds and how to treat them. This 17 page parchment is unique among the remaining papyri of the time (Ebers Papyrus and London-Leiden Medical Papyrus) because of its rational and scientific approach. The other papyri were medical texts based on magic.

Imhotep, who was the architect of the step pyramid at Saqqara, would have seen many cases of broken bones and men injuring themselves by falling while building this large structure. While dealing largely with trauma and surgery, the Smith Papyrus was highly descriptive. Forty-eight specific cases are documented. Examples include: "Instructions Concerning a Wound on the Top of His Eyebrow." After this follows the details on the examination of the patient and a diagnosis. Bob Brier also notes: "Here the physician is told to state the injury and then whether or not he can treat it" [3]. Actually, there were three things he could say: (1) "An ailment which I will treat"; (2) "An ailment with which I will contend"; and (3) "An ailment not to be treated." In these writings we see the concept of prognosis as well as treatment. Egyptian physicians also described diseases which were beyond treatment as "an affliction for which nothing can be done." For example, the surgical portion was the first of its kind revealing a methodical identification of an ailment starting from the top of the head and working downward. The development of methods would be a theme encouraged by Sir William Osler centuries later.

Details on closing wounds with sutures, preventing and curing infection with honey, and recommendations to immobilize those with head and spinal cord injury as well as other lower body fractures are described. Physicians used bandages, splints, plaster, tape, and sutures. They also advised suppositories, herbal dressings, enemas, and castor oil. Gold was used to bind teeth and facial abscesses were incised and drained. Aloe vera was used for skin disease.

The first translation of the Smith Papyrus was by James Henry Breasted. This translation revealed that rational, scientific practices were based on careful observation and examination. While many of the treatments used in ancient Egypt are now considered to be of little benefit, some approaches set the bar for the art of medicine as we know it today. Imhotep's work formed a basis for how to care for the patient. Hippocrates and Galen, both of whom studied Egyptian works, would later acknowledge his contribution.

Hammurabi

Freedom from disease is the first blessing

—Siddartha Gotama

Reverence for good health has been documented since the beginning of recorded history. Siddartha Gotama (563 BCE–483 BCE), the great spiritual leader from India and the founder of Buddhism, inscribed his philosophies on the importance of good health as far back as 500 BCE. Historically, many cultures have allowed the medical practitioner to enjoy a distinguished—even holy—place in society, respected in the same manner as spiritual or religious leaders and philosophers. Medicine is one of the greatest vocations to which a person can devote his or her life. It creates opportunity for individuals to provide service to society as healers, teachers, and respected role models. Many cultures recognize the special and complex part medical practitioners play in directly affecting the health of their people. Physicians are rewarded for a job well done, yet are held responsible when their work is acknowledged or perceived as less than satisfactory. This theme has threaded itself throughout time, with origins as far back as known recorded history.

Societies have held physicians accountable for their conduct since well before the time of sixth Babylonian King Hammurabi (ca. 1795–1750 BCE). The *Code of Hammurabi* represents perhaps one of the earliest of recorded laws, consisting of a total of 282 edicts carved into a 6-ft tall stone monument for all to see. Prominently displayed is the code of patient care, which reads:

> If a physician make a large incision with an operating knife and cure it, or if he open a tumor (over the eye) with an operating knife, and saves the eye, he shall receive ten shekels in money ... If a physician heals the broken bone or diseased soft part of a man, the patient shall pay the physician five shekels in money. [4]

This concept rings true to the modern understanding of the physician–patient interaction. A health service is provided and upon completion the physician is compensated. Today there are many expectations about what constitutes a successful interaction, which stem from both objective rules of proper procedure established by decades of scientific research and subjective ideals, values, and thoughts unique to each patient. Completing an "unsuccessful" health encounter certainly has consequences today; however, if you did harm in the era of the Babylonian empire, you would suffer an extremely severe punishment. Also included in Hammurabi's rules are the consequences for an unsatisfactory job:

> If a physician makes a large incision with an operating knife, and kills him, or opens a tumor with an operating knife, and cuts out the eye, his hands shall be cut off ... [4]

Whether we like it or not, society continues to hold us accountable for all interpretations of unsuccessful care. Of course, avoiding mutilation or reprimand is not why we want to be excellent healers; however, current thoughts about punishment or consequences for a physician who has not fulfilled his or her expectations often echo this sentiment. It is important to remember that we have been granted special rights by the people whom we serve. We are fiduciaries to a wealth of knowledge, services, and information that will directly affect our patients' health, and because of this we wield an incredible power. How do we harness and channel this power toward the good of our patients?

In this book, we will look at some of the earliest lessons of the art of medicine, handed down by teachers from as far back as more than a century ago. We are privileged to make our way down a road that is well traveled by those who have come before us, those who have learned the intricate and sometimes obscure secrets of patient care. To begin this story, we must start with the Greeks.

Hippocrates

> Medicine is of all the Arts the most noble; but, owing to the ignorance of those who practice it, and of those who, inconsiderately, form a judgment of them, it is at present behind all the arts [5]
>
> —Hippocrates (460 BCE–ca.370)

Even 2000 years ago, physicians struggled to learn about the *art* of medicine, and philosophers contributed much to its interpretation. Although he is highly recognized as the Father of Medicine, little is known about Hippocrates of Cos, also known as Hippocrates the Great (460 BCE–?356) (see Fig. 2.1). "All we know about Hippocrates is legend," notes Roy Porter in *The Greatest Benefit to Mankind* [6]. Two hundred years after his death, the Greeks founded the Library of Alexandria with the aim to compile and organize thousands of medical writings provided by many medical, religious, and spiritual philosophers. Works attributed to Hippocrates stood out for the detailed nature in which the author described those suffering from diseases. All writings that seemed to follow this unique style were thereafter noted as having been written by Hippocrates and represent the Corpus Hippocraticum—the bodies of work that followed his distinguished theories about health and humanity. Although all of the texts of the Corpus Hippocraticum follow his spoken philosophies and detailed style of analysis, experts agree that many of the works attributed to this collection were certainly not penned by Hippocrates [5].

One of the most frequently cited English translations of Hippocratic texts was written by the Scottish surgeon Francis Adams in 1849 [5]. The reader is referred to this text to learn more about the veracity of different treatises ascribed to Hippocrates. Suffice it to say that for the remainder of the discussion on Hippocrates I will refer to these writings as being by Hippocrates, with the understanding that it cannot be proven that he actually wrote what has been attributed to him.

Throughout my career, the majority of medical students I have encountered are unable to cite much more about Hippocrates than the famously quoted "Primum non nocere," or "First do no harm." If you had to remember only one line attributed to Hippocrates, this is undoubtedly the most important one to remember. It is a theme that spans the entirety of medical practice; yet there is so much more that is learned from Hippocrates as one explores his life, personal experiences, and teachings.

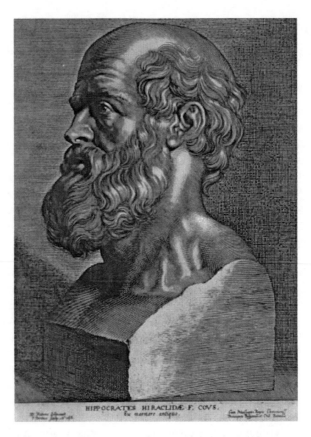

HIPPOCRATES HIRACLIDÆ F. COVS.
In marmore antiquo.

Fig. 2.1 Hippocrates (Engraving by Peter Paul Rubens, 1638, courtesy of the National Library of Medicine, accessed from http://www.encyclopedia.com/topic/Hippocrates.aspx)

Hippocrates was renowned for his power of observation, thought by many to be his greatest skill. His followers were known for practicing bedside medicine. In a collection of his writings entitled *Aphorisms,* there are over 200 observations of medical practice, disease process, and pathological theory [5]. Many of these are still relevant today, and those that are not as applicable to modern medical practice are of great interest as they provide insight into the evolution of medicine. Furthermore, although some of his conclusions have been shown to be made without current standards of scientific validation, it is important to recognize the value Hippocrates placed on the physician's skill of observation and its application to the patient. This is as important today as it was over two millennia ago. A few of Hippocrates' observations from *Aphorisms* follow:

1. Life is short and the art long, the occasion fleeting, experience fallacious, and judgment difficult. The physician must not only be prepared to do what is right himself but also to make the patient, the attendants, and externals cooperate.
2. For extreme diseases, extreme methods of cure, as to restrictions, are most suitable.
3. Spontaneous lassitude indicates disease.
4. Persons who are naturally fat are apt to die earlier than those who are slender.
5. In whatever part of the body heat or cold is seated, there is disease.
6. If erysipelas of the womb seizes a woman with child, it will probably prove fatal.
7. Pneumonia coming on pleurisy is bad.
8. Delirium upon division of the cranium, if it penetrates into the cavity of the head, is bad.
9. When bubbles settle on the surface of urine, they indicate disease of the kidneys and that the complaint will be protracted.
10. Sleep and watchfulness, both of them when immoderate, constitute disease.

Some aphorisms may make you laugh, such as

1. Drinking strong wine cures hunger.
2. If you wish to stop the menses in a woman, apply as large a cupping instrument as possible to the breasts.
3. A woman does not become ambidextrous.
4. Eunuchs do not take the gout nor become bald.

The requirement for careful observation was greatly impressed upon me as a medical student. I clearly remember lessons such as whenever you visit a patient in the hospital you should not leave without paying close attention to the surroundings. It is important to notice even such seemingly plain facts as what objects are on the patient's bedside table, which friends and family members have or have not come to visit, or the name of the medication label on the intravenous bag. You just might discover something that will help you understand and know your patient better, shed light on unique attitudes and expectations, or simply enable you to more effectively care for this patient. The skill of observation is one that I emphasize to my current medical students as much as possible.

I once entered the room of an African-American gentleman who was admitted the previous night suffering from chest pain. At his bedside sat a book describing the inequality that exists in health care delivery to minorities. It reminded me that many members of our society experience health care disparities and, moreover, that this subject was something my patient thought very important. For me to gain the confidence of this particular patient, I knew that I would need to clearly communicate my plan to provide him with the best health care and to follow through on this expectation as well. Sometimes by looking at more than the physical patient you will observe factors which will help you help the patient. This can remind you of something profound: that your patient is a complex individual with a unique cultural, social, and religious background. Or it may be something as simple—but equally as important—as finding out that your patient is not receiving the medication you ordered. Given that a 2006 Institute of Medicine report noted that over 1.5 million adverse drug events occur in the USA each year due to physicians' oversight is an additional reason to be observant [7]. Yogi Berra once said, "You can observe a lot by just watching." All healers do this; some do it better than others.

Some simple but critical observations you do not want to miss include such details as the pack of cigarettes in your patient's pocket, how your patient just crossed her arms as you gave advice she disagrees with and how this may negatively affect her compliance, and the atypical skin lesion which catches your eye as you listen to your patient's posterior thorax. Another subtle observation not to be missed might include the slight change in mental status of an elderly patient, potentially denoting an early sign of sepsis or dementia. When I was a third-year medical student, one professor explained to me, "The organs of the aged do not cry out in pain." I have remembered this throughout my years of clinical practice and it has served me well. Observe all.

Hippocrates cautioned that we evaluate *honestly*. The fact that physicians of his time were observed as being less than honest speaks of the human frailties to which we are all susceptible. We have all heard stories or perhaps been witness to physicians who do not evaluate honestly. The Hippocratic Oath, recited by most medical students prior to graduation, urges physicians to act in a professional manner and not provide therapy for our patients for personal financial gain. "I will not cut persons laboring under the stone but will leave this to be done by those who are practitioners of this work," Hippocrates wrote in *The Oath* [5]. Many occupations refer to themselves as "professional," but this term takes on a very complex meaning when it is used to denote a physician, dentist, nurse, or other health practitioner. Below is a definition of the professional, as described by a rising third-year student in response to her University of Maryland School of Medicine's application essay prompt:

> Entering a profession implies embracing every aspect of a practice through diligence and devotion, that motivates one to develop their skills in an area of academia in order to grow as an individual; moreover, to use this growth as a means to satisfactorily provide a service to their community. A professional is someone who has worked rigorously to learn their craft, and loyally dedicates their time and effort to perfecting it; yet at the same time realizes that perfection is not easily attainable, nor is it guaranteed. Nonetheless, they pursue the goal of professional and self-fulfillment through constant intellectual, spiritual and self-actualizing growth. Their profession is constantly progressing and expanding and is interdisciplinary in the knowledge, social, and communicatory skills needed to effectively impact its seekers. Entering into a profession is not a simple proclamation of what one is going to accomplish. Rather, it is an embarkation that wholly encompasses every aspect of that person. It is a declaration of where one's future will take them and, most importantly, the efforts to make this possible through important life choices and significant dedication to those choices. Entering into a profession is an exciting journey, a life-changing commitment to service that will better one's community. Not only this, but it is entry into a greater, more expansive domain of professionals. A profession cannot exist through the efforts of just one person, and entering into one must also convey the professional's understanding and embracing of the need to work with others in order to have a successful and respected career. Entering a profession is the first step toward one's fulfilling career in providing a necessary service to society and the greater human good [8].

In the healing arts, the practical and simplified definition of professionalism implies that the professional will follow a course of action that is best for the patient, even at the expense of what may be best financially or personally for him- or herself. The commitment to this notion is symbolically conveyed by recitation of the Hippocratic Oath upon graduation from medical school. Many non-physicians are at least superficially familiar with the Hippocratic Oath, likely because of the great importance it represents not just to physicians but to the public we serve. The Hippocratic Oath follows:

The Hippocratic Oath [5]

I swear by Apollo the physician, and Aesculapius, and Health, and 7All-heal, and all the gods and goddesses, that, according to my ability and judgment, I will keep this Oath and this stipulation—to reckon him who taught me this Art equally dear to me as my parents, to share my substances with him, and relieve his necessities if required; to look upon his offspring in the same footing as my own brother, and to teach them this art, if they shall wish to learn it, without fee or stipulation; and that by precept, lecture, and every other mode of instruction, I will impart a knowledge of the Arts to my own sons, and those of my teacher, and to disciples bound by a stipulation and oath according to the law of medicine, but to none others. I will follow that system of regimen which, according to my ability and judgment, I consider for the benefit of my patients, and abstain from whatever is deleterious and mischievous. I will give no deadly medicine to any one if asked, nor suggest any such counsel; and in like manner I will not give to a woman a pessary to produce abortion. With purity and holiness I will pass my life and practice my Art. I will not cut persons laboring under the stone, but will leave this to be done by men who are practitioners of this work. Into whatever house I enter, I will go into them for the benefit of the sick, and will abstain from every voluntary act of mischief and corruption; and further, from the seduction of female or males, or freemen and slaves. Whatever, in connection with my professional practice or not, in connection with it, I see or hear, in the life of men, which ought not to be spoken of abroad, I will not divulge, as reckoning that all such should be kept secret. While I continue to keep this Oath unviolated, may it be granted to me to enjoy life and the practice of the art, respectful by all men, in all times! But should I trespass and violate this Oath, may the reverse be my lot!

The Hippocratic Oath expresses many significant concepts regarding health and health care expectations. It is interesting to reflect upon the issues that were felt to be important over two millennia ago and moreover, to recognize that many of these remain controversial in modern times. Clearly these were considered critical and honorable notions at the time of its creation. Have they evolved to mean something different over the centuries? Or are we, as physicians, still learning them?

The idea that physicians should practice beneficently and do what is best for their patients is truly a recurring theme in medicine and society and it will surface many times in this book. This concept is certainly not contentious, but as we will see it is felt by several teachers in the current century to be in need of reiteration. Euthanasia and abortion were clearly concepts about which Hippocrates felt strongly. Throughout the centuries, these topics evoke strong emotions from both patient and health care provider and continue to polarize many people in medicine, politics, religion, and society. It is up to physicians to sort through their own values on these controversial subjects and decide their practices accordingly. This is followed in the oath by a declaration that as healers we should live a life of purity and holiness. From this interpretation it almost sounds like we are entering a religious order, yet the fact that the healer's examining room is often likened to a confessional strengthens this notion. It may be a stretch to compare practicing physicians to priests; however, in both instances those seeking service divulge the innermost secrets about their bodies and personal lives to a trustworthy advisor. Both physicians and religious figures are healers of people, and like priests, rabbis, and teachers we share a common vocation to serve society.

Passion follows next in the Hippocratic Oath. While it is important to show compassion for our patients, Hippocrates notes it is not appropriate to be passionate with our patients. Unfortunately throughout the USA and the world of medicine, there continues to be reports of physicians who engage in inappropriate relationships with their patients. It is beyond the scope of this book to discuss in detail what may or may not represent an inappropriate relationship or to impose certain morals or excuse exceptional situations. Suffice it to say that the American Psychiatric Association has decreed that a sexual relationship with any patient, past, present, or future, is not advised. It is important to remember that although both physician and patient are human, protocol and professional expectation creates boundaries that must be followed to provide unbiased and effective care.

Perhaps one of the most important notions emphasized in the oath is that of physician–patient confidentiality. The Hippocratic Oath reminds us that we should not divulge what we have learned from our patients. Our communications and patient interactions must be kept secret in order to maintain patient trust, safety, and dignity, and to uphold the protocol established by past professionals. In the USA, the recently enacted Health Insurance Privacy and Portability Act (HIPPA) governmental laws serve to emphasize this point. HIPPA was enacted by the United States Congress in 1996. The privacy rule took effect on April 14, 2003 and regulates the use and disclosure of protected health information, including the medical record, by health care providers. Someone faithful to the Hippocratic Oath, with goals of maintaining professionalism and upholding the written laws surrounding the consequences of digression, will not divulge any details of one patient's care to another who did not have consent or the express need to know.

The temptation to break this ethic can be subtle and seemingly innocent. An example that I will never forget occurred when one of my patients let me know that her best friend, also one of my patients, was not doing well. She requested that I contact her friend to check in. After what seemed like a minute or two, I did not reply to her. When she asked me specifically what I was going to do about this situation I told her, "I cannot discuss with you whether I do or do not see Mrs. _____. If she were a patient of mine, I would not be at liberty to speak to another person about her care." The concerned friend under my immediate care became livid in the exam room, raised her voice, and stormed out of the office. She angrily pointed a finger at me as she left and threatened, "If anything happens to her, I will hold you responsible." This situation is a dramatic example, but it illustrates the importance of upholding your standards for all patients, even if they are close friends or family. A much less spectacular example of this is the time I bumped into a patient in the grocery store. After a friendly greeting, he told me that his boss, also my patient, spoke with him about a recent visit to my office. I think you can guess my reply. It may seem overprotective, but it is important to keep in mind that even the most innocent or seemingly benign invitations to divulge knowledge about another patient must be respectfully declined. This must be done in such a manner that you do not infer that, yes, you did see this patient. To do so without consent would not be professional or legal.

Porter notes, "The art of diagnosis involved creating a profile of the patient's way of life, habitation, work, and dietary habits" [9]. Hippocrates urged that when it comes to therapeutics we should "assist nature" [5]. He strongly advocated the encouragement of patients to take better care of themselves by changing their lifestyles, particularly when it came to following a prescribed diet: "A slender and restricted diet is always dangerous in chronic diseases." Likewise, Hippocrates advocated exercise or activity for certain ailments: "It should be kept in mind that exercise strengthens, and inactivity weakens" [5]. Although many of his prescriptions would now be viewed as ludicrous by today's standards, his concern for well-being is parallel to current medical practice's mindfulness of the importance of diet, exercise, and activity with regard to patients' health. In recent years, this concept has become more applicable with the overwhelming surge of metabolic syndrome diagnosis, childhood and adult onset diabetes, obesity, coronary artery disease, hypertension, and many other preventable health problems currently plaguing our country.

According to Hippocrates, one of the important qualities for a physician to cultivate is the ability to prognosticate:

> For by foreseeing and foretelling, in the presence of the sick, the present, the past, and the future, and explaining the omissions which patients have been guilty of, he will be the more readily believed to be acquainted with the circumstances of the sick; so that men will have confidence to entrust themselves to such a physician ... He will manage the cure best who has foreseen what is to happen from the present state of matters [5].

In the *Book of Prognostics* (ca. 400 BCE) we also learn one way in which Hippocrates avoided the malpractice of his day—*censure* [5]. This implies that by being aware of the natural history of a disease and whether or not medical intervention will indeed improve a condition, the physician would best be able to counsel a patient about what to expect in the course and outcome of their illness. In the age of Hippocrates, it was recognized that effective communication between physician and patient was one of the best ways to avoid censure, particularly in matters when the prognosis was poor. Honest information about what the patient should or should not expect regarding his or her illness was as important then as it is now. Not only does it base the patient's apprehensions in reality, but it also allows for informed decision-making of both parties involved. Furthermore, it strengthens the physician–patient relationship as the patient's trust in his or her doctor is reaffirmed.

In acute diseases the physician should first observe the "countenance" of the patient. Hippocrates compiled some prognostic indications of a poor patient outcome, which are still recognized as valid. These are listed below:

- Hollow eyes
- Collapsed temple
- Cold ears
- A black, green, livid (black and blue; deathly colored), or lead-colored face

[The above four are part of the *facies hippocratica* or the facial look of dying]

- Seeing the whites of patients' eyes when they are sleeping
- Cold sweats to the head, face, or neck (these in acute fever prognosticate death)

- A swelling in the hypochondria (the area that is just underneath the anterior rib cage, to the left and right of the epigastrium bilaterally) that is hard or painful
- All dropsied (disease with drops, or water, edema, e.g., congestive heart failure) arising from acute diseases is bad
- It is a bad symptom when the head, hands, and feet are cold while the belly and sides are hot
- Strong and continued headaches with fever, if any of the deadly symptoms be joined to them, are very fatal

Others of his prognostics are not as applicable to medical practice today and may be placed under the category of just plain funny, such as

- It is best when wind passes without noise, but it is better that flatulence should pass even thus than it should be retained

Hippocrates' teachings have stood centuries of scrutiny. In this section, we have only briefly reviewed a few of his lessons. Lessons from the Father of Medicine that still are applicable to the physician of today are many. Some of the most important lessons I think the reader should learn from Hippocrates follow: first do no harm, observe all, evaluate honestly, prognosticate when you can and when it comes to therapeutics, and assist nature. Additionally, healers of any era should recognize that we are not in the practice of medicine for money but to serve our fellow man, and that we would be wise to learn from our predecessors in medicine and by carefully studying our patients. Lastly, it is ideal that we should live our life with purity and holiness as we practice our art. Hopefully I have generated an interest in you to read more about the Father of Medicine and the Corpus Hippocraticum. But there are other Greeks we have to discuss!

Early Greeks

An incredible part of what we have come to understand as being important to the practice of medicine came from an era when not only Hippocrates but also Aristotle, Socrates, and Plato taught their philosophies.[1] Many students complain about the tortuous and

---

[1]As with Hippocrates, the mention of these contributors is unfortunately brief and focuses only on illuminating some of the basics of the art of medicine.

unpleasant experience of being asked esoteric questions for which the answers are known largely by a more educated senior group. This ritual has even evolved its own derogatory name: "pimping." Interestingly, this style of teaching is similar to the Socratic dialogue, attributed to the classical Greek philosopher Socrates (469 BCE–399 BCE). Put simply, it involves teaching a student by asking questions, such that the student's answers will lead to further questions. This lends itself to understand a greater truth or a more complex lesson.

Much of what is known about Socrates comes from the writings of Plato. From the treatise *The Charmides*, a conversation between Socrates and a young boy, we learn of the importance of temperance. This is a very significant lesson in medicine; in fact, it provides the foundation upon which medicinal practice is built. Medicine is derived from Indo-European *med-*, to take appropriate measures [10]. From the Latin *mederi*—to look after, heal, and cure—stemmed the words medicine and remedy. Other derivatives led to the words *modern*, *modest*, and *moderate*. Being appropriately moderate may well be one way in which a healer can best practice his or her art. Patients from antiquity to the current day do not always welcome our efforts to look after them. Alexander the Great reportedly exclaimed on his death bed, "I die by the help of too many physicians." This sentiment is shared by Miquel de Cervantes in Don Quixote when the Padre hopes that doctors looking to cure a mad man are successful: "May it not be worse than the disease" [11]. We are urged by Socrates to be temperate, and as healers we can sometimes do the best for our patients by doing the least. As physicians, we become true practitioners of the healing art when we recognize the potential for illness and disease to improve naturally with time and overcome the urge to provide unnecessary physiological therapy. Surgeons in particular are aware of this, the best of whom help their patients by declining an opportunity to operate in instances when they know it will not benefit the patient.

The word doctor is derived from the Indo-European root *dek* (to take, to accept) via the Latin *docere*, to teach [10]. It is critical to the physician–patient relationship that we understand the impact and power of our ability to teach our patients. It is too often overlooked. An important lesson for the young healer is to recognize that often it is not "the pill in the hand, but the hand behind the pill" that helps our patients feel better [12]. It is important that we educate our patients about their health so that they may better take care of themselves. A 1998 survey looking at prescription of antimicrobials highlighted this concept. In evaluating attitudes of parents and physicians concerning the prescribing of antimicrobials to a pediatric population, 65% of patients expected to receive an antibiotic for treatment of an upper respiratory infection [13]. In this study there was no correlation between patient satisfaction and receipt of an antibiotic prescription [13]. Instead, patient satisfaction correlated highest with the quality of the physician–patient interaction. Results from focus groups indicate that patients would be satisfied if an antibiotic was not prescribed as long as the physician explained the reasons for the decision to withhold antibiotics [13]. It has also been shown that patients who are informed have lower anxiety and complication rates compared to those who are uninformed [14–17]. This is *docere* in action!

Another important art we can cultivate in our office visit is to consider asking our patients if there is anything about their illness that particularly concerns them. Many patients fear that the symptom they are experiencing may represent something terrible or fatal, which may in fact not be the case at all. Reassurance that in your experience a certain symptom is not at all likely to cause a certain terrible outcome is sometimes the major agenda our patients have in making an appointment to see us, even if this concern is not clearly communicated. Other patients focus on what may seem to us as mundane or simple worries, but addressing these concerns may make all the difference in the patient's personal interpretation of the health care encounter, its effectiveness, its success, and your abilities as a physician. Being a good prognosticator is truly valued.

During the office visit, it is our responsibility to teach our patients what they can do to take better care of themselves. This may entail specific and clear recommendations about diet, exercise, social habits, such as smoking and drinking, or other activities. An excellent way to open the discussion toward teaching your patients is to simply ask them at the end of your visit, "Do you have any questions for me?" We should be clear in giving our opinion as to when they should return in follow-up—be it as needed, in 3 months, if condition worsens, etc.— and must strive to set reasonable health goals *with* our patients to emphasize the partnership we are forming to improve their health. Understanding that we are teachers is critical to mastering the healer's art. From the root *dek-* of the Latin word *docere* also comes the word *discere*, to learn, from which we get the current derivation *disciple* [10]. *Dignity* and *decent* are also derived from the same Indo-European root. As doctors we are our patients' teachers and must provide them with the environment to learn so as to better their physical and mental wellness. Hippocrates teaches us to be a student of nature, life, and illness by observing all. Others have described this full circle of education by saying, "A good teacher is a good student first." [18]

References

1. Osler W. Project Gutenberg's the evolution of modern medicine, by William Osler. The evolution of modern medicine a series of lectures delivered at Yale University on the Silliman Foundation in April 1913. New Haven, CT: Yale University Press; 1921. Release Date: February 21, 2006 [EBook #1566].
2. http://www.crystalinks.com/egyptmedicine.html. Accessed Jun 2012.
3. Brier B. Ancient Egyptian magic. New York: William Morrow; 1998.
4. King LW. The code of Hammurabi, vol 22. Whitefish, MT: Kessinger Publishing; 1910. p. 215–21. Trans. L.W. King.
5. Adams F. The genuine works of hippocrates, vol 2. New York: W. Wood and company; 1886. p. 283. Trans. F. Adams.
6. Porter R. The greatest benefit to mankind. New York: W.W. Norton & Co; 1997.
7. Institute of Medicine, Preventing medication errors, report brief, Jul 2006. http://www.iom.edu/File.aspx?ID=35943. Accessed May 2009
8. University of Maryland School of Medicine Class of 2011 Admission Essay provided by Caitlin E. Iafolla Zaner.
9. Livingstone RW editor. The legacy of GREECE, essays by Murray G, Inge WR, Burnet J, Heath Sir TL, Thompson D'Arcy W, Singer C, Livingston RW, Toynbee A, Zimmern AE, Gardner P, Blomfield Sir R. Oxford: The Clarendon Press; Aug 6, 2007. http://www.mlahanas.de/Greeks/Texts/Books/MedicinePart.html. Accessed 2012. Printed in England at the University Press, by John Johnson Printer to the University
10. Houghton Mifflin Company. The american heritage dictionary of the English language. 4th ed. Wilmington, DE: Houghton Mifflin Company; 2000.
11. Quixote D, De Cervantes M. A New Translation by Edith Grossman, Harper Perennial; Reprint edition (April 26, 2005).
12. Anonymous.
13. Barden LS, et al. Current attitudes regarding use of antimicrobial agents: results from physician's and parents' focus group discussion. Clin Pediatr. 1998;37:665–71.
14. Cabot R. The use of truth and falsehood in medicine, an experimental study. In: Reiser S et al., editors. Ethics in medicine. Cambridge: MIT Press; 1977. p. 213–20. Reprinted.
15. Hooker HW. Truth in our intercourse with the sick. In: Reiser S et al., editors. Ethics in medicine. Cambridge: MIT Press; 1977. p. 206–12.
16. Kant I. Ethical duties towards others: truth-fullness, in his Lectures on Ethics. New York: Harper Torchbooks; 1963. p. 224–34.
17. Oken D. What to tell cancer patients. In: Gorovitz S et al., editors. Moral problems in medicine. Englewood Cliffs, NJ: Prentice-Hall; 1970. p. 109–15.
18. Soni MK. 2012. http://www.wow4u.com/mksoni2/index.html. Accessed Jun 2012.

Imhotep

Osler W. The Silliman Foundation of modern medicine: a series of lectures delivered at Yale University on the Silliman Foundation in April 1913. New Haven, CT: Yale University Press; 1921.

Brier B. Ancient Egyptian magic. New York: William Morrow; 1998.

Osler W. The evolution of modern medicine. Whitefish, MT: Kessinger Publishing; 2004. p. 12.

Highfield R. How Imhotep give us medicine, The daily telegraph. www. Telegraph.co.uk. Accessed Mon 10 Oct 2011

Mostafa Shehata MD. The father of medicine: a historical reconsideration. J Med Ethics. 2004;12:171–6.

Dunn J. Imhotep, Doctor, Architect, High Priest, Scribe and Vizier to King Djoser. http://touregypt.net/featurestories/imhotep.htm. Accessed 10 Oct 2011

http://www.crystalinks.com/egyptmedicine.html

Hammurabi

King LW. The code of Hammurabi, vol 22. Whitefish, MT: Kessinger Publishing; 1910. p. 215–21. Trans. L.W. King.

Van De Mieroop M. King Hammurabi of Babylon: a biography. Oxford: Blackwell Publishing; 2005.

Siddartha

Hesse H. Siddartha. Los Angeles, CA: Norilana Books; 2007.

Hippocrates

Adams F. The genuine works of Hippocrates. Baltimore, MD: Williams & Wilkins Co; 1939. Trans. F. Adams.

Jacques J. Hippocrates: medicine and culture. Baltimore, MD: The Johns Hopkins University Press; 1998. Trans. M. DeBovoise.

Potter P. Loeb classical library: Hippocrates, vol. 5. Cambridge, MA: Harvard University Press; 1988.

Lloyd G. Hippocratic Writings. New York: Penguin Classics; 1950. Trans. J. Chadwick.

Early Greeks

Longrigg J. Greek medicine from the heroic to the Hellenistic age: a source-book. London: Duckworth Publishing; 1977.
Sigerist H. A history of medicine, vol. I and II: early Greek, Hindu, and Persian medicine. Oxford: Oxford University Press; 1961.

History of Medicine

Porter R. The greatest benefit to mankind. New York: W.W. Norton & Co; 1997.

Chapter 3
Chinese and Medieval Medicine

Three Divine Doctors of Jian An

This text is not offered up as a history of medicine tome, but rather a guide to help the healer learn more about the art of caring. Chinese Medicine can proudly point to the lives of the Three Divine Doctors of Jian An as being exemplary in showing care for others.

From the perspective of Dr. Marta Hanson, Professor of History of Medicine at Johns Hopkins University, the accounts of the Three Divine Doctors of Jian An are more literary and mythological than historical. Dr. Hanson notes "Nonetheless it is still worthwhile to look at the lives of these three physicians since even as mythic figures they have had a great deal of influence on ideas of how physicians should behave morally. Although based on historical figures, these three physicians have become mythologized to represent morally exemplary physicians" (Personal communication).

Zhang Zhongjing

Zhang Zhongjing (150–219 AD) is considered to be one of the greatest Chinese physicians in history and well known to those practicing modern Chinese medicine, yet very little is known about him. He learned medicine by studying from a local mentor, reviewing the medical literature available at that time, and gleaning the prescribing habits of others far and wide. His major work, "Treatise on Cold Pathogenic and

R. Colgan, *Advice to the Healer: On the Art of Caring*,
DOI 10.1007/978-1-4614-5170-9_3,
© Springer Science+Business Media, LLC 2013

Miscellaneous Diseases," was lost during the many wars that took place in the era of the Three Kingdoms (220–280 AD).

Zhang made great contributions to traditional Chinese medicine including "On Cold Damage," which revealed how to treat rampant epidemic fevers, and "Essential Prescriptions of the Golden Coffer," an overview of his clinical observations. The latter was written some 700 years earlier than the Arabic physician Avicenna's *Canon of Medicine*. Zhang's book contained over 100 typical prescriptions and close to 400 curative methods and disease postulates for which many of today's traditional Chinese medicine treatment principles are derived. An interesting observation attributed to Zhang has some relevance even today perhaps:

> In terms of the high level, medicine is for curing nobles of their diseases; in terms of the lower level, it is used to save the poor from disaster; in terms of the middle level, it is used to keep us in good health [1].

Zhang Zhongjing, like other ancient traditional Chinese medicine doctors, viewed being a physician as a sacred privilege as opposed to an occupation. Even though Zhongjing was promoted to a high municipal office as recognition of his worth, he continued to see patients while practicing his official duties. His commitment to serving others was so profound that he resigned his position as Governor of Changsa when those around him criticized him for attempting to do both, rather than give up his care for his patients.

Hua Tuo

Hua Tuo (ca. 140–208) lived during the late Han Dynasty and Three Kingdoms era. Hua Tuo is described in the *Book of Later Han* as the first Chinese physician to use anesthesia. By using combinations of wine, herbs, and narcotics, patients were made intoxicated (if not insensate) which allowed for surgery. Fan's biography of Hua Tuo lists medical cases that spanned internal medicine, surgery, gynecology and pediatrics [2]. He reportedly treated ulcers and sores, performed abortions, and removed parasites. Hua Tuo was also popular for promoting disease prevention and recommending that people exercise to strengthen their health. Hippocrates would later take up this same cause. Hua Tuo developed the "Exercise of the Five Animals," incorporating differing types of body movements imitating movements of the tiger, deer, bear, monkey, and crane.

Hua Tuo is one of the "Three Divine Doctors in Jian An" who was committed to his patients and considered medicine a higher calling. He turned down being a military officer several times so as to follow medicine. He would later lose his life for this belief. Hua Tuo successfully cared for the government leader of the day, Cao Cao, who was demanding and frequently ordered Hua Tuo to attend to him. On one occasion Hua Tuo stood his ground and made excuse after excuse, replying that he could not come right away as he had to attend to matters at home. His failure to return when summoned led to him being brought to Cao Cao against his will, imprisoned and put to death for his insubordination.

Dong Feng

Dong Feng rounds out the list of the "Three Divine Doctors of Jian An," and he is the reason I chose to add Chinese medicine to this second edition. I include him because of the great compassion and love he showed for his patients, and even more, however, he is included because of his acknowledgement of the importance of caring for the community at large, particularly those who could not afford medical care.

Dong Feng reportedly enjoyed equal fame to Zhang Zhangjing and Hua Tuo and was a highly skilled doctor in the era of the Three Kingdoms as well. He practiced medicine in the Lushan Mountains where his skill and deeds became legend. He treated his patients but did not charge them a fee. If he cured someone with a serious illness he asked them to plant five apricot trees on the mountain slope. If he cured someone of a general illness, he would ask them to plant one tree. Because of his fame, people came from far distances to be cared for by him and over time the apricot trees became a forest with many thousands of trees. He reportedly posted a sign that read: "Those who want to buy apricots do not need to tell me, but could just leave a liter of rice in exchange for a liter of apricots" [3]. The rice that was exchanged for apricots helped those who were having financial difficulties or refugees fleeing famine. Dong Feng is credited with having saved and helped over 20,000 people in his lifetime. People later came to refer to traditional Chinese medicine as "Apricot Tree Forest." He was so beloved that upon his death people built an apricot altar for him. Apricot trees still grow in the place where Dong Feng practiced medicine 1800 years ago.

The Three Doctors of the Divine Era were learned, wise, and caring healers who showed the art of caring by serving others without consideration for their own personal gain or welfare. They realized that what they were doing was more important than who they were. Learning what they could from those who came before them, using whatever resources they had at hand, and being mindful that each person has within themselves resources for self-betterment was important. Lastly, we have seen from Chinese medicine that the health of the individual and the health of one's community are both to be cherished.

Rhazes

Abu Bakr Muhammad ibn Zakariya Razi (865 ACE–ca. 923 ACE) was one of the greatest physicians of the Middle Ages (see Fig. 3.1). Known as Rhazes, this man was regarded as an influential alchemist,

Fig. 3.1 Rhazes (pictured at the bedside of a young patient afflicted with measles. Accessed from http://dodd.cmcvellore.ac.in/hom/09%20-%20Rhazes.jpg)

philosopher, and Persian scholar. Like so many of the great physicians we will discuss in this book, Rhazes was known not only for what he contributed to the art of medicine, but for his commitment to scholarly work as well.

Historically, Rhazes is remembered for numerous writings on medicine, including pediatrics, ophthalmology, neurosurgery, and pharmacy. A prolific author of his time, he published books and articles in the disciplines of alchemy, religion, and philosophy as well. He is perhaps best known for having authored a nine-volume compendium entitled *Continens Liber* or *The Large Comprehensive*. But the focus of this book is to highlight the contributions which the greatest teachers of medicine and other healing arts have given us as they apply directly to the physician–patient relationship. In short: How is it that we — as clinicians — come to regard a specific behavior or style of practice as exemplary? Who can we look to as a role model? Who are the icons that have shown themselves as masters of the art of caring, specifically as it pertains to the physician–patient relationship? How do we know a great healer when we see one? Rhazes helped us to understand by example what we now recognize as superb practice.

Rhazes, like Imhotep and Hippocrates, advocated for use of the power of observation, and in doing so he encouraged scientific inquiry in caring for the patient. Since the time of Hippocrates, the humoral theory was held by physicians as the basis for their understanding of disease. According to Galen of Pergamum, a prominent philosopher of Greek origin, a person was sick if one of their four humors — black bile, yellow bile, phlegm, and blood — were out of balance. Humoralism was closely linked to the Greeks' theory of four elements — earth, wind, fire, and water. By observing his patients in a specific and particular manner, Rhazes challenged the notions of those before him. He was the first to refute the opinions of Galen in *Doubts About Galen*, which ultimately led to the dismissal of humoralism as nonscientific. This change in thinking did not occur quickly, and Rhazes was met with much resistance for many years. In fact, his thinking was not fully accepted until Rudolph Virchow developed his thesis on cellular pathology in the mid-nineteenth century.

Rhazes urged practitioners to think independently and to learn from their experiences with disease through meticulous observation and constant questioning. Using these practices himself, he published some of the first scientific descriptions of medical illnesses, and he is even credited with providing the first accounts of such diseases as smallpox and measles. Rhazes also disagreed with Galen over the nature of fever and urinary ailments, basing his opinions on his own practice and patient observations. He taught, "All that is written in books is worth much less than the experience of a wise doctor" [4]. Living by his own lessons led him to many discoveries. He was the first to describe allergic rhinitis and asthma in a scientific manner. His writing *A Dissertation on the Cause of the Coryza (acute inflammation of the mucous membranes of the nasal cavities) which Occurs in the Spring When the Roses Give Forth Their Scent* is the first known publication on hay fever.

Rhazes advocated for the practice of evidence-based medicine in the Middle Ages. He developed standards of question and practice that provided the foundation for modern thought on evidence-based medicine, which few physicians would argue against today. Rhazes taught that physicians should look at whether or not a disease was curable versus non-curable with implication of multiple treatments; further, they should use the information gained to change their practices for the betterment of the patient. When it came to caring for those with cancer and leprosy, Rhazes urged that the physician not be blamed for his patient's poor outcome. He was a fierce independent thinker who, while urging diligent study and the pursuit of knowledge, also taught humility and caution when it comes to unrealistic expectations of being confident in what we seemingly know. He taught that "truth in medicine is an unattainable goal, and the art as described in books is far beneath the knowledge of an experienced and thoughtful physician" [5].

In addition to promoting the skills of observation and independent thinking, Rhazes argued that we should be ethical and moral about our daily routine:

> The doctor's aim is to do good, even to our enemies, so much more to our friends, and my profession forbids us to do harm to our kindred, as it is instituted for the benefit and welfare of the human race, and God imposed on physicians the oath not to compose mortiferous remedies [5].

Although he was a physician to the rich and powerful, Rhazes' devotion to medical education and treatment of the poor made him highly sought after as a teacher by medical students of his day. Rhazes was known for treating the impoverished sick free of charge during a time when medical care by physicians of such repute was mainly enjoyed by those of wealth. He pioneered the teaching of medicine by the bedside, and also wrote a self-help home remedy guide for the common man after recognizing that many could not afford to seek professional medical care.

Rhazes possessed the wise and insightful thought that physicians should be mindful of their patients' mental health just as well as their physical health. He wrote of the importance of a sound mind and a sound body and discussed the significant positive impact afforded to those physicians humble enough to be friendly with their patients. He has been called "probably the greatest and most original of all Muslim physicians" [6]. Rhazes was known as much for his intelligence as for his kindness and compassion to others. He was troubled by poverty and suffering and gave away his fortune, such that he died in destitution.

Avicenna

Another Persian teacher of medicine was the physician and philosopher Abu Ali Sinna (980 ACE–1037 ACE) (see Fig. 3.2). Also known as Hakim Ibn Sina, he is more commonly known in the West as Avicenna. Avicenna is known as the father of early modern medicine. Like many of the great teachers we discuss in this book, he is known by those outside of medicine for many significant accomplishments. And like other medical giants he was a prolific writer, with hundreds of treatises still in existence. Avicenna's best-known works are *The Book of Healing* and the 14-volume *Qanun* or *Canon of Medicine*. Completed in 1025 ACE, it served as a foundation for medical teaching for over 700 years. *The Canon of Medicine* is considered by many to represent the first pharmacopeia, including more than 600 medicinals, chemicals, and physical properties and details of their implementation. Avicenna also wrote of the necessity of studying drugs before exposing them to the public, antedating our current practice of clinical trials by hundreds of years. Avicenna was recognized by Osler as "author of the most famous medical textbook ever written" [7]. He noted that Avicenna's *Canon* remained "a medical bible for a longer time than any other work" [7]. Copies of an English translation can still be purchased and are the basis for modern-day primary medical pharmaceutical texts.

Fig. 3.2 Ibn Sina or Avicenna (public domain)

Like many of the great healers already discussed, Avicenna is known for promoting the power of observation and experimentation. He practiced evidence-based medicine and helped elucidate the contagious nature of infectious disease, introducing the concept of quarantine (forty days) to control outbreaks of infections. He cared for the sick—often at no cost—brought to him in great numbers because of his renowned reputation. Avicenna's contribution to the art of medicine may be that he was a thinker, scholar, and someone adept in the intellectual pursuit of diverse topics that affect mankind. In addition, he incorporated thoughts and ideas from those who preceded him, which helped shape his own growth in many disciplines. Avicenna was influenced by Hippocrates, Aristotle, Galen, Rhazes, and Indian medicine. This becomes a recurring theme of the great healers: looking to the teachings of others before them for guidance and knowledge in how they should proceed in the practice of their art.

Avicenna incorporated physical, emotional, and spiritual medicine into his system of healing. Like Rhazes, Avicenna also recognized that emotional illness could be expressed in physical complaints. In the *Canon* he describes an illness afflicting a prince, which puzzled the local doctors for its severity but apparent lack of physical cause. Avicenna noted a fluttering in the prince's pulse whenever the name or address of his love interest, from whom he was separated, was mentioned. The patient was promptly cured upon being reunited with his lover. Avicenna, like many of the great physicians discussed in this book, was able to recognize that patients complaining of physical symptoms can have an underlying emotional discord as the cause for their discomfort. The ability to rule out organicity and diagnose a patient with a functional disorder is a hallmark of a great healer. This ancient doctor of doctors was a champion for the use of herbals and dietary changes to promote wellness. Like Hippocrates (and many of our mothers), he believed that food was the best medicine. Most of us can surely relate to the admonitions of "Doctor Mom," who extols the virtues of chicken soup, carrots, spinach, and other foods as being good for us.

Avicenna was able to incorporate what he had learned from others into a way of caring for his patients that was best suited for each individual. He promoted scientific study and careful detailing of the medical and pharmaceutical procedures he used on his patients. Further, he used these principles for those who could and could not afford his services and donated his time and efforts to help underserved and impoverished populations. For those he could not directly care for, he offered assistance by developing manuals of health care for the layperson. This is how Avicenna continues to teach us today. He reminds us to look back to our ancestors and learn from them to create new knowledge in a scientific manner and to use the information gained to reach out and heal our current patients.

Maimonides

Moses Maimonides (1135 ACE–1204 ACE), also known as Rabbi Moshe ben Maimun or Rambam was perhaps the most famous Jewish physician in Arabic medicine (see Fig. 3.3). Born in Cordova, he later migrated to Palestine and then to Cairo to avoid religious persecution. This rabbi, philosopher, scholar, and writer is revered by those of the

Fig. 3.3 Moses Maimonides (Portrait, nineteenth century, author unknown. Commonly used image indicating one artist's conception of Maimonides's appearance, accessed fromhttp://commons.wikimedia.org/wiki/File:Maimonides-2.jpg)

Judaic faith, not because of his stature as physician, but as one of their greatest theologians. As one of my medical students, who is an observant Jew told me, "When we think of Maimonides, his role as a physician is about eighth down on the list of what he is known for in Judaism." Maimonides wrote a number of texts, including *Fusul Musa* or *Chapter of Moses*, a collection of medical aphorisms. When researching the long list of those who should be considered in a text about the art of medicine as taught by the masters of medical education, Maimonides name is immediately thrust to the top of this list because of his devotion to his patients and his passion for service.

Maimonides was the physician to a sultan, and in a letter sent to Samuel (Shmuel) ibn Tibbon he described the typical scene that awaited him at home after a long and brutal day of work:

> I would find the antechambers filled with people, both Jews and Gentiles, nobles and common people, judges and bailiffs, friends and foes — a mixed multitude, who await the time of my return. I dismount from my animal, wash my hands, go forth to my patients, and entreat them to bear with me while I partake of some slight refreshment, the only meal I take in

the 24 hours. Then I attend to my patients, and write prescriptions and directions for their various ailments. Patients go in and out until nightfall, and sometimes even, I solemnly assure you, until 2 hours and more in the night. I converse with and prescribe for them while lying down from sheer fatigue, and when night falls I am so exhausted that I can scarcely speak ... I have here related to you only a part of what you would see if you were to visit me [8].

With regard to the physician–patient relationship, Maimonides' true greatness manifested as a complete commitment to his patients. One can picture this weary man stumbling into his home only to find, amidst the hanging lanterns and dim light, mothers holding their sick children with looks of fear on their faces. Interestingly, Maimonides refers to his practice as *healing*. If you will remember, so did Hammurabi. Maimonides revered the great teachers of medicine who preceded him and singled out Hippocrates as "Head of Physicians." Like Hippocrates, Maimonides taught students of medicine, and advocated that "a physician should begin with simple treatment, trying to cure by hygiene and diet before he administers drugs." Recognizing the lessons of those who come before us is characteristic of many of the physician-teachers highlighted in this book. As Maimonides looked back to Hippocrates for inspiration, so too did Osler look back to Maimonides for his wisdom and highly regarded the Jewish scholar as the "Prince of Physicians."

Maimonides possessed love for his profession, a true dedication to his practice and his patient. He recognized his skill as a gift from God and passionately wrote of this realization. He is thought by some to have expressed these thoughts in *The Physician's Oath and Prayer*. Although the authorship of this text by Maimonides has been called into serious question—it is felt by others to be the work of Markus Herz (1747–1803), a German physician and pupil of Immanuel Kant—this does not detract from the beauty of what follows:

The Physician's Oath and Prayer of Maimonides

The Oath of Maimonides

The eternal providence has appointed me to watch over the life and health of Thy creatures. May the love for my art actuate me at all times; may neither avarice nor miserliness, nor thirst for glory or for a great reputation engage my mind; for the enemies of truth and philanthropy could easily deceive me and make me forgetful of my lofty aim of doing good to Thy children.

May I never see in the patient anything but a fellow creature in pain. Grant me the strength, time and opportunity always to correct what I have acquired, always to extend its domain; for knowledge is immense and the spirit of man can extend indefinitely to enrich itself daily with new requirements.

Today he can discover his errors of yesterday and tomorrow he can obtain a new light on what he thinks himself sure of today. Oh, God, Thou has appointed me to watch over the life and death of Thy creatures; here am I ready for my vocation and now I turn unto my calling [9].

The Prayer of Maimonides

"Almighty God, Thou has created the human body with infinite wisdom. Ten thousand times ten thousand organs hast Thou combined in it that act unceasingly and harmoniously to preserve the whole in all its beauty the body which is the envelope of the immortal soul. They are ever acting in perfect order, agreement and accord. Yet, when the frailty of matter or the unbridling of passions deranges this order or interrupts this accord, then forces clash and the body crumbles into the primal dust from which it came. Thou sendest to man diseases as beneficent messengers to foretell approaching danger and to urge him to avert it.

Thou has blest Thine earth, Thy rivers and Thy mountains with healing substances; they enable Thy creatures to alleviate their sufferings and to heal their illnesses. Thou hast endowed man with the wisdom to relieve the suffering of his brother, to recognize his disorders, to extract the healing substances, to discover their powers and to prepare and to apply them to suit every ill. In Thine Eternal Providence Thou hast chosen me to watch over the life and health of Thy creatures. I am now about to apply myself to the duties of my profession. Support me, Almighty God, in these great labors that they may benefit mankind, for without Thy help not even the least thing will succeed.

Inspire me with love for my art and for Thy creatures. Do not allow thirst for profit, ambition for renown and admiration, to interfere with my profession, for these are the enemies of truth and of love for mankind and they can lead astray in the great task of attending to the welfare of Thy creatures. Preserve the strength of my body and of my soul that they ever be ready to cheerfully help and support rich and poor, good and bad, enemy as well as friend. In the sufferer let me see only the human being. Illumine my mind that it recognize what presents itself and that it may comprehend what is absent or hidden. Let it not fail to see what is visible, but do not permit it to arrogate to itself the power to see what cannot be seen, for delicate and indefinite are the bounds of the great art of caring for the lives and health of Thy creatures. Let me never be absent-minded. May no strange thoughts divert my attention at the bedside of the sick, or disturb my mind in its silent labors, for great and sacred are the thoughtful deliberations required to preserve the lives and health of Thy creatures.

Grant that my patients have confidence in me and my art and follow my directions and my counsel. Remove from their midst all charlatans and the whole host of officious relatives and know-all nurses, cruel people who arrogantly frustrate the wisest purposes of our art and often lead Thy creatures to their death.

Should those who are wiser than I wish to improve and instruct me, let my soul gratefully follow their guidance; for vast is the extent of our art. Should conceited fools, however, censure me, then let love for my profession steel me against them, so that I remain steadfast without regard for age, for reputation, or for honor, because surrender would bring to Thy creatures sickness and death.

Imbue my soul with gentleness and calmness when older colleagues, proud of their age, wish to displace me or to scorn me or disdainfully to teach me. May even this be of advantage to me, for they know many things of which I am ignorant, but let not their arrogance give me pain. For they are old and old age is not master of the passions. I also hope to attain old age upon this earth, before Thee, Almighty God!

Let me be contented in everything except in the great science of my profession. Never allow the thought to arise in me that I have attained to sufficient knowledge, but vouchsafe to me the strength, the leisure and the ambition ever to extend my knowledge. For art is great, but the mind of man is ever expanding.

Almighty God! Thou hast chosen me in Thy mercy to watch over the life and death of Thy creatures. I now apply myself to my profession. Support me in this great task so that it may benefit mankind, for without Thy help not even the least thing will succeed."

In the *Oath of Maimonides* he cites, "Here am I ready for my vocation and now I turn unto my calling." This is one of the earliest times in recorded history that we see the field of medicine being referred to as a vocation and a calling. It is clear that Maimonides viewed his work as a physician as sacred, given to him by God so that he could help his fellow man. Indeed, Maimonides states, "Providence Thou hast chosen me to watch over the life and health of Thy creatures." What inspirational words! I do not imagine there is a single reader who feels differently about his *art*. History has noted the greatness of Maimonides for his contributions to religion and philosophy, more so than his contributions to medicine. His service to his people, patients, and students is undeniable in many disciplines. That he inspired others to think led to the Jewish adage about him, attributed to the German–Jewish Philosopher Moses Mendelssohn (1729–1786):

"From Moses unto Moses there arose not one like Moses [10]." We are truly fortunate that a healer as devoted and humanistic as Maimonides found an intellectual and spiritual outlet in medicine.

References

1. www.chinaculture.org/gb/en_aboutchina/20003-09/24/content_26689.htm
2. medlibrary.org/medwiki/Hua_Tuo
3. http://www.pureinsight.org/node/1368
4. http://www.bookrags.com/biography/abu-bakr-muhammad-ibn-zakariya-ar-razi-woh/
5. Islamic science, the scholar and ethics. FCTC Limited 24 Feb 2006. 1 May 2009. http://www.muslimheritage.com/topics/default.cfm?ArticleID=570
6. Browne EG. Islamic medicine. Delhi: Goodword Books Pvt. Ltd.; 2001.
7. Osler W. The evolution of modern science. New Haven, CT: Yale University Press; 1921. p. 243.
8. Illievitz AB. Maimonides the physician. Responsa Pe'er HaDor. Can Med Assoc J. 1935;32:440–2.
9. Friedenwald H. Bull Johns Hopkins Hosp. 1917;28:260–1.
10. Chapters on Jewish Literature, Israel Abrahams, Chapter XIII. Moses maimonides. May 2009. http://www.authorama.com/chapters-on-jewish-literature-13.html

Three Divine Physicians of Jian An

Wai FK. On Hua Tuo's position in the history of Chinese medicine. Am J Chinese Med. 2004;32(2):313–20.
DeWoskin KJ. Doctors, diviners and magician's of ancient China: biographies of Fang-shih. New York: Columbia University Press; 1983.
Association for Asian Research. Hua Tuo: a miraculous healer in ancient China. http://www.asianresearch.org/articles/895.html
Zhang Zhongjing. China culture http://www.chinaculture.org/gb/en_aboutchina/2003-09

Rhazes

Stolyarov G II. Rhazes: the thinking western physician. The Rational Argumentator. 2002; Issue VI. http://www.liberalinstitute.com/IslamicPhysicianRhazes.html
Ranking GSA. The life and works of Rhazes. In Proceedings of the seventeenth International Congress of Medicine; London; 1913. p. 237–268

Avicenna

Gordon D, Christensen L, Dayrit M, Dela F, Karle H, Mercer H. Educating health professionals: the avicenna project. Lancet. 2008;371(9617):966–7.

Goodman LE. Avicenna. London: Taylor and Francis; 2003.

Browne E. Islamic medicine. Dehli: Goodword Publishing; 2002.

Maimonides

Kraemer J. Maimonides: the life and world of one of civilizations greatest minds. New York: Doubleday; 2008.

The Maimonides Heritage Foundation. Maimonides, a biography. 2005. 20 Feb 2009. http://www.maimonidesheritage.org/History.asp

Chapter 4
The Twentieth Century

Florence Nightingale[1]

I always feel as if God had said: Mankind is to create mankind.

–Florence Nightingale

If asked to identify one woman throughout history whose name is synonymous with providing care to the sick, most people would likely answer: Florence Nightingale. A British nurse, pioneer of modern nursing, public health advocate, and noted statistician, Nightingale (1820–1910) dedicated her life to serving others (see Fig. 4.1). The story of Florence Nightingale must be told in a book which looks to provide advice to clinicians on the art of caring. She truly stands out as one of the greatest healers history has known.

Florence Nightingale was born in Italy into a well-to-do English family. Her parents named her after the city where she was born. Her family members were land owners, developers of mines and quarries, farmers, bankers, and members of parliament. Nightingale was raised in privilege, at a time when few women chose professions or social causes. She cared little for socializing ("a waste of time") or suitors. Nightingale was born into a family where she was expected to live a life of gentility, yet such comforts meant nothing to her. From her teenage years until her twenties, she cared for people from nearby villages who worked or lived on her family's estates. Serving many,

---

[1] Written with Deborah Ann Colgan, R.N.

R. Colgan, *Advice to the Healer: On the Art of Caring*,
DOI 10.1007/978-1-4614-5170-9_4,
© Springer Science+Business Media, LLC 2013

she worked long hours without rest. Her father questioned her actions and asked why she did not act like other women who married and had a family. Her reply was forthright: "Father, the strong do not need my help. They can take care of themselves. I believe in doing religion, not talking it" [1]. Florence was deeply religious, deriving strength from doing God's work and caring for mankind. She honed these skills in serving British soldiers during the Crimean War. At a time when bureaucracy and red tape was rampant in the Department of War, she fought for the basic necessities for her country's men in battle. "Save these soldiers' lives and then talk army regulations," she said. "Give me blankets, food, medicine. Give me more help. I do not care for your systems and regulations, but I do care for the wounded and the sick" [1]. Spending her own money on supplies, she would make nightly rounds on the sick, with her lantern in her hand to light the way. According to one historian of the day, "she finally made the British soldiers of the Crimea healthier than the civilian population of England" [1]. She earned the reputation for being a genius of organization, likely due in part to her sense of extreme confidence that she could accomplish most anything she set her mind to.

Upon her return from war, a great reception awaited "the lady with the lamp" and her shipmates. As the boat approached the dock on the Thames River, rather than accept the applause which was sure to be heard, she slipped away from the boat and quietly found her way to her home in London (and went to bed) rather than accept applause and attention on the dock. Thereafter, she used her organizational and networking skills to identify how she might bring the greatest good to the most people. She also used the knowledge she gained from the battlefields of the Crimea to pioneer the modern hospital. What we find commonplace in most hospitals today, she championed in London in 1856.

Nursing historian Barbara Montgomery Dossey's comprehensive text *Florence Nightingale Today* attributes the following list of accomplishments to her: the Pavilion system of buildings, isolation of communicable diseases, personal comforts for patients, cleanliness to an extreme degree, and the well-trained nurse [2]. Dossey notes in this text, "Both the patients' internal and external environment was viewed by Nightingale to be important. This included their bed and bedding, food, light, the patients' cleanliness as well as that of the room." Nightingale taught her nurses to avoid unnecessary noise, as well to not give false hope, promises, or advice. She had a holistic

Fig. 4.1 Florence Nightingale (circa 1860) in shawl. This is the preferred image of her by her family [Florence Nightingale (1820–1910) ca.1860 (b/w photo), English Photographer, (nineteenth century)/British Library, London, UK/© British Library Board. All Rights Reserved/The Bridgeman Art Library]

perspective to include not only mind, body, and biosocial but the spiritual element of each patient as well. This advice need not apply to just nurses.

Before the bacterial origin of infectious disease was known, at a time when bacteria were killing more people than those dying on the battlefields, Florence Nightingale fought for improved sanitation and the conversion of hospitals from "pesthouses" to wards with proper sanitary conditions. "It may seem a strange principle to enunciate as the very first requirement in a hospital that it should do the sick no harm" [3], she noted. In *Notes on Nursing*, she identified the following five items as being important to the "health of houses": pure air, pure water, efficient drainage, cleanliness, and light. Nightingale advocated for "total healing environments" [4]. This entails observing the patients' problems and managing well their care. She also

promoted cleanliness and how to avoid disease outside of the
hospital. She worked to develop uniform systems for hospital statistics as well as disease classification. She created a novel pie chart like
descriptor, the Coxcomb diagram, to present statistics in a clearer
manner. Working with William Farr, the founder of medical statistics,
she created applied statistical tables listing the numbers of soldiers
who had died, where they had died, and their cause of death. Using
these tools, she was able to show that in peacetime, English soldiers
were twice as likely to die compared to the rate of civilians. Because
of this work, she is credited with persuading Queen Victoria of the
need to improve sanitary conditions in military hospitals. Her contributions to public sanitation, public health, and statistics are beyond
the scope of this book yet are some of her greatest accomplishments.
We mention them here to highlight her far-reaching efforts to improve
the human condition.

A working premise of this book is that clinicians in the caring
professions can learn from others outside of their own respective
discipline. Physicians, dentists, and pharmacists can learn from
nurses, social workers, and psychologists. To do so, we must recognize the value each contributes in caring for the total patient and
believe that together we function best as a team. Some of the lessons
taught by Florence Nightingale on how to care for the patient are
worth noting because we can modify them to our own respective
disciplines. To follow are some specifics on the art of caring as taught
by this matriarch of nursing.

Florence Nightingale's Notes on Nursing Which Apply to the Art of Caring

Observe the sick.
Never let a patient be waked out of his sleep.
Avoid unnecessary noise: Whisper outside the room.
View and sunlight are matters of first importance to the sick.
Leading questions are useless or misleading.
Obtain accurate information[2].

---

[2] Nightingale tells the story of a "clever" physician who began taking a history of
those with abdominal pain with the question "point your finger where you be bad."

Be confidential.

Children are much more susceptible than grown people to noxious influences[3].

Florence Nightingale, a woman of small stature and sick much of her life, was a visionary leader and a great healer. She was periodically confined to bed rest during the Crimean war yet would not let this deter her from helping the English troops. These soldiers were so touched by her dedication that they had to be given turns in sharing the privilege of carrying the "Lady-in-Chief" from hospital to hospital on a stretcher. She is described by the British physician and biographer Mosby as a rugged individual, not in stature but in her spirit and courage [1].

Nightingale was chosen to exemplify the art of caring for many reasons. She was a selfless nurse who realized that the only thing that mattered was the patient. She fought stereotypes and societal pressure and identified what was needed, both on the battlefield and in the City of London. She then committed herself to improving the public's health. Like many of the great healers described in this book, she is remembered more than one hundred years after her death for how she lived her life. Like Avicenna, Nightingale was someone who took care of patients, one at a time, while appreciating the importance of caring for the masses. Like Maimonides, she referred to her vocation as a calling and worked tirelessly. Like Schweitzer, she dedicated her life to service because of a conviction that it was how to best serve God. Dossey notes, "To Nightingale, nursing was service to God and service to humanity. She believed that the aim of human life was to create heaven here and now on earth" [2].

Medical historian Dr. Phillip Mackowiak offers the possibility that her periods of boundless energy alternating with extreme fatigue which caused her to "take to the bed" might have been due to post-traumatic stress disorder after returning from the Crimea. A cogent argument is also made for the possibility that she also suffered from what is now called bipolar disorder [5].

Florence Nightingale died at the age of 90. While the exact cause of her death has been debated, her death certificate lists old age and heart failure.

---

[3] "They are affected by the same things, but much more quickly and seriously."

Nightingale turned down an offer of burial at Westminster Abby. Instead, it was her wish that she have a quiet burial and be interred next to her father and mother at Embley with the simple inscription "F.N." on her tombstone.

Santa Filomena

–by Henry Wadsworth Longfellow

Whene'er a noble deed is wrought,
Whene'er is spoken a noble thought,
Our hearts, in glad surprise,
To higher levels rise.
The tidal wave of deeper souls
Into our inmost being rolls,
And lifts us unawares
Out of all meaner cares.

Honor to those whose words or deeds
Thus help us in our daily needs,
And by their overflow
Raise us from what is low!

Thus thought I, as by night I read
Of the great army of the dead,
The trenches cold and damp,
The starved and frozen camp,--

The wounded from the battle-plain,
In dreary hospitals of pain,
The cheerless corridors,
The cold and stony floors.

Lo! in that house of misery
A lady with a lamp I see
Pass through the glimmering gloom,
And flit from room to room.

And slow, as in a dream of bliss,
The speechless sufferer turns to kiss
Her shadow, as it falls
Upon the darkening walls.

As if a door in heaven should be
Opened, and then closed suddenly,
The vision came and went,
The light shone was spent.

On England's annals, through the long
Hereafter of her speech and song,

That light its rays shall cast
From portals of the past.

A lady with a lamp shall stand
In the great history of the land,
A noble type of good,
Heroic womanhood.

Nor even shall be wanting here
The palm, the lily, and the spear,
The symbols that of yore
Saint Filomena bore.

Sir William Osler

To prevent disease, to relieve suffering and to heal the sick- this is our work.

–Sir William Osler

One of the most influential English-speaking physicians in history was the Canadian medical educator Sir William Osler (1849–1919). Following postgraduate training in England and Europe, he taught medicine and pathology at many institutions including McGill and the University of Pennsylvania and, in 1889, was the first professor of medicine at Johns Hopkins University. In 1905, Osler became Regius Professor of Medicine at Oxford. Sir William Osler's impact on medical education is likely far greater than any other teacher in the history of Western medicine.

Osler is considered the *father* of internal medicine and authored the textbook *The Principles and Practice of Medicine* in 1892, which was widely used for decades. This text inspired John D. Rockefeller to establish the Rockefeller Institute for Medical Research. Osler's description of infectious endocarditis led to his name being associated with infectious nodules—painful, purple, and on the palm and the soles of afflicted patients (Osler's nodes). But Osler's greatest legacy was as a medical educator. He pioneered the concept of teaching students by having them learn directly from patients. At a time in history when students were largely taught only in classrooms, he championed the concept of gathering knowledge at the bedside. Osler wrote, "He who studies medicine without books sails an uncharted sea, but he who studies medicine without patients does not go to sea at all" [6].

Osler prided himself in his role as a medical professor. He was once quoted, "On my epitaph I would like nothing else written other than ... 'he taught medical students in the wards,' for I view this by

far as the single greatest thing I have ever done" [7]. It is clear that
Osler contributed greatly to the science of medicine, lending more
documented detail on physiology and disease process than perhaps
anyone before him. So what did he have to offer with regard to the art
of medicine? Osler indoctrinated two cardinal concepts to his students that every physician should have (1) *imperturbability* and (2)
aequanimaty:

> Imperturbability means coolness and presence of mind under all circum-
> stances, calmness amid storm, clearness of judgment in moments of grave
> peril, immobility, passiveness ... and the physician who has the misfortune
> to be without, who betrays indecision and worry, and who shows that he is
> flustered and flurried in ordinary circumstances, loses rapidly the
> confidence of patients [6].

Imperturbability comes from wide experience and a deep understanding of the subject matter. Of this notion Osler wrote, "No quality
takes higher rank" [6]. He recognized education, practice, and experience would help the student to develop this skill.

I remember a classic example of a young physician, only a year
out of medical school, who did *not* showcase his imperturbability in
a time of crisis. As a medical student, I observed this new physician
called onto the wards to attend to a patient suffering from shock. The
patient was with altered mental status, hypotension, and near cardiac
arrest. The intern, who to his defense had no desire whatsoever to be
a somatic physician, rushed out of the room chaotically. Obviously
flustered, waving his arms frantically he shouted to the nurse,
"Someone call a doctor!" The grounded nurse replied, "You are a
doctor!" Ultimately, a "code blue" was called, and the patient was
transferred to the coronary care unit. I am certain that to this day, the
intern, now a practicing psychiatrist, is thankful that he is far away
from the medical wards. The notion of imperturbability is also
described in the aphorism "the first pulse you should take in a code
is your own." In other words, when faced with an emergency, check
yourself to be sure that you are not overreacting or flustered, before
looking to render aid. This is easier said than done, particularly for
young healers. But do not despair over being of a young age. Osler
also felt that "the real work of life is done before the 40th year and
that after the 60th year it would be best for the world and best for
themselves if men rested from their labours" [8].

According to Osler, an important accompaniment to imperturbability is aequanimaty, defined as the mental embodiment of imperturbability. An example cited in a collection of Osler's works

entitled *Aequanimatus* is the physician's ability to bear, with composure, the misfortune of others. For some, this may come as a natural skill. For others, it must be learned. Being patient with those who might not have attained your level of knowledge or experience is a display of aequanimaty. Inherent in this concept is the fact that absolute truth is unattainable and that we must be content in our knowledge that in so many situations in medicine—and in life—we do not hold all the pieces of the puzzle.

This brings me to a critical concept for the young healer. All physicians learn clinical medicine in the wards and in outpatient clerkships. Some students prefer to gather knowledge about clinical medical practice and procedure from readings and lectures. This is essential. Yet most experienced clinicians will tell you that their greatest lessons were taught by preceptors in a clinical setting, as both student and teacher partnered together in caring for a patient. This mentoring is critical in the maturation process of the future physician and provides valuable insight on interactions between different levels of authority, responsibility, and experience in the delivery of health care. Unfortunately, I have never met a medical student who (when asked) did not admit to having been derided or mocked on occasion during this process. The following account of my first clinical rotation in medical school illustrates this point well:

> I was excited to be a third year student in the emergency department of a large county hospital after my basic science curriculum, during which I had little clinical exposure. Amid one memorable shift, I was in the process of learning how to change a Foley catheter when the senior resident interrupted my tutorial and yelled aloud to the other staff, "He has no pulse … CODE BLUE!" To my shock the patient was quickly wheeled from underneath my arms to the cardiac arrest area of the emergency room. The ER attending, Dr. Melvin Sharoky, with aequanimaty and imperturbability called for more information about the patient. I tried to speak, but no words escaped until seemingly minutes later when I blurted out, "Schneiderman and Berard." The intern David Schneiderman and medical resident Michael Berard were quickly summoned and assisted as the attending ("one who attends") ran the code. I stood there helplessly, intensely watching the passing of a human life. Then the code was over. Dr. Sharoky said, "I'm calling it," and our patient was pronounced dead.

> As is the custom after a cardiac arrest, physicians will pause and discuss the case to try to learn from it—to figure out if something could have been done differently. The ER attending physician was asked, "What do you think killed the patient?"

> He replied, "I'll tell you what I think killed the patient. I think the medical student killed him by pulling on the Foley catheter."

> I was stunned. It was my first real memory of being involved in the care of a patient, and I'd heard from the senior physician that I killed a man.

But he was not serious. This was a teaching point, not a true indictment. The lesson was that manipulation of a catheter in a gravely ill man—albeit often necessary—has the potential to induce a vagal response, i.e., the patient's heart rate can decrease, which may be the touché that forces life to leave a man's body. I later learned that our patient died of pneumococcal sepsis and meningitis, a deadly disease, which few escape. But this wise ER attending's teaching point will never leave me: Be careful. Another lesson might have been that junior clinicians must get used to taking feedback from their superiors, so as to learn how to practice great medicine. In this setting, as a third year student, I didn't know any better and thought that these comments were meant as a true measure of inadequacy of my involvement in this case. I now know it was not, and that we must accept all types of criticism, lessons, and even sarcasm delivered so as to learn how to care for our patients.

The aforementioned scenario was an example of clinical medical education delivered with good intentions. Learning clinical pearls in academia is not always wrapped in niceties. Sometimes students rightfully perceive that a lesson is being taught in less than a good-spirited manner. To the young healer, I urge you to not let a colleague or senior teacher put you down or make you feel small for not knowing something. You have either witnessed or seen it happen, I am sure. For example, a student is asked, "What are the five most common types of lymphoma?" to which he replies in exasperation "I don't know … I only know two: Hodgkins and Non-Hodgkins!" This is followed by the smug teacher slowly walking away with a smirk and a sense of false victory. Pity these educators for they do not have the knowledge to know that they make themselves inferior, not superior, by attempting to put you down. In fact, I believe that one of the smartest answers to any question is, "I don't know … but I will look it up and get back to you." Pity any hubristic colleague who might attempt to disrespect you in such a way and then teach them.

It is in this area that Osler was truly a giant. In his work *Teacher and Student*, Osler lists four characteristics which each student should strive for [9]. The first is the "art of detachment" or being mindful to properly balance work and play. This is not to suggest that students should not enjoy themselves but rather that we should show self-control in pursuing our delights and not allow ourselves to be overly attached to certain frivolous attractions. Osler urges that we develop a discipline of self-control so that we may live laborious days.

Second is the "virtue of method." Osler cites the efficiency of the successful businessman, who owes part of his success to the fact that he has developed a systematic and an orderly arrangement to his work. The best medical students and physicians I have worked with have figured this out. Some carry a notebook with them to keep track of ideas; others keep a log of outstanding tests they have ordered but have not seen the results return yet. We healers must practice medicine under the guidelines of established system and method. In other words, get into the habit of doing the same thing every time, so that certain behaviors become your usual and customary practice. An example of this follows: Every time a patient tells you he/she has a fever, your method should be to follow this up with the question, "How high?" If he/she reports the fever to be in the truly febrile range, for example, over 100 °F, your method should be to inquire if he/she had chills. And if chills are noted—again—your method should dictate you to ask, "Are these shaking chills … bed rattling or teeth chattering chills?" These qualities denote rigors, a possible indicator that the patient is suffering from what may potentially be a life-threatening bacteremia. In such instances, the bacterial cell wall components are perceived as foreign by the thermoregulatory center of the brain, which responds through a cascade of signals causing the body to shake vigorously. This is an example of a good method every healer may care to follow in addressing a patient with fever. It represents a straightforward but complete process that will most efficiently lead to diagnosis and most importantly save your patient's life.

Another example of good method can be practiced every time you write a prescription. Consider lifting your head up as your pen is touching the prescription pad and ask, "Are you allergic to anything?" This simple question can quickly become extremely important if its answer is missed or overlooked. The reason being that preventable medication errors occur frequently and the last thing you (or your patients for that matter) want is the occurrence of a frightening allergic reaction on top of their current ailments. One of the greatest errors which we are responsible for is the inappropriate prescribing of a medication to a patient. According to the Institute of Medicine, up to

25% of inpatients receive an incorrect medicine during their hospital stay [10]. A similar example occurs with regard to magnetic resonance imaging (MRI) scans and metal objects. It will do you well to look up each time you write an order for an MRI scan and ask your patient, "Do you have any metal inside you?" It is another simple question and often your patients will require further explanation, "Yes that includes piercings, pins, pacemakers, tattoos ... " Unfortunately, patients have been harmed by physicians ordering an MRI without checking for metal objects. They learn this as the patient is injured during what should be a routine procedure, as the metallic particles are pulled to the surface. Sticking to this methodical series of questioning will avoid potentially uncomfortable and painful situations for those under your care.

Third is the quality of "thoroughness," knowledge of the fundamental science on which medicine is based. Osler encouraged students to write down their notes and to not trust their memory. We should "observe, record, tabulate and communicate" and "use (our) five senses" to accomplish thoroughness (see Figs. 4.2, 4.3, 4.4 and 4.5). We are urged to be aware of these idealistic principles and not just attend to the minuscule details of chemistry, anatomy, and physiology. We are urged to avoid charlatanism and fraud and to study diligently the fundamentals of our discipline, so as to be truly prepared to care for our patients. A great healer, at a minimum, should be competent.

With this competence must also exist the "grace of humility," the recognition that we are capable of personal error and cannot always be right; moreover, at some point, we are simply going to be wrong. With every occupation come risks and consequences. If we are wrong as bakers, we may burn our rolls. But as healers, our mistakes carry a significant chance that great harm may come to our patients. An anonymous quote explains the serious truth that often, "Lawyers hang their mistakes. Journalists put their mistakes on the front page. Doctors bury their mistakes." Patients will die because of our mistakes, some of which may be preventable. It is our goal as healers to uphold the positive qualities explained by those before us to minimize this occurrence and to learn from any misfortune so as to prevent its reoccurrence. Osler gives advice on this as well:

> ... Errors in judgment must occur in the practice of an art which consists largely of balancing probabilities. Start, I say, with this attitude in mind, and mistakes will be acknowledged and regretted, but instead of a slow

Fig. 4.2 Sir William Osler inspection (Courtesy of Pamela Miller, History of Medicine Librarian, Osler Library of the History of Medicine, McGill University, Montreal, Quebec Canada. Used with permission)

process of self-deception, with ever-increasing inability to recognize truth, you will draw from your errors the very lessons which may enable you to avoid their repetition [9].

An excellent read on the life of Sir William Osler can be found in Charles S Bryan's *Osler: Inspirations from a Great Physician*. Bryan has divided this book into chapters whose titles alone describe important lessons for every young healer. I have chosen to highlight several chapters below along with some of the more salient take home points, as I see them [11].

Fig. 4.3 Sir William Osler auscultation (Courtesy of Pamela Miller, History of Medicine Librarian, Osler Library of the History of Medicine, McGill University, Montreal, Quebec Canada. Used with permission)

Manage Time Well: Day-Tight Compartment

Osler urged that we be methodical and plan each day with definite goals in mind. He taught a concept called "day-tight compartments" best summarized as not concerning ourselves with the past or the future but rather focusing on the present. His method was to set aside specific hours of each day for writing, while being sure that he also had time for his interpersonal relationships. Osler believed that "punctuality is the prime essential of a physician- if invariably on time he will succeed even in the face of professional mediocrity" [12]. Dr. Harvey Cushing, (1869–1939), the renowned American

Fig. 4.4 Sir William palpation (Courtesy of Pamela Miller, History of Medicine Librarian, Osler Library of the History of Medicine, McGill University, Montreal, Quebec Canada. Used with permission)

neurosurgeon and a biographer of Sir William Osler, was impressed with how he made time to read and write and yet still had time for other things which were viewed as important, such as writing an obituary for a friend or taking a medical student he had not seen for years to lunch. "He knew how to capture the moment" [13].

Osler admired a poem written sometime around 400 AD by an Indian dramatist named Kalidassa. This poem follows.

Listen to the Exhortation of the Dawn!
Look to this Day
For it is Life, the very Life of Life.
For Yesterday is but a Dream
And Tomorrow is only a Vision;

Fig. 4.5 Sir William contemplation (Courtesy of Pamela Miller, History of Medicine Librarian, Osler Library of the History of Medicine, McGill University, Montreal, Quebec Canada. Used with permission)

But Today well lived makes
Every Yesterday a Dream of Happiness,
And every Tomorrow a Vision of Hope.
Look well therefore to this Day!
Such is the Salutation of the Dawn!

Find a Calling: Being True to Certain Ideals

Osler enrolled for a short time at Trinity College in Toronto thinking he would enter the ministry before making up his mind to pursue medicine. Even after he was well established, he was urged to consider other paths, such as university president and politician, but he declined. In perhaps his greatest speech to a medical student body, titled Aequanimatus, he spoke of having found his "calling":

To prevent disease, to relieve suffering and to heal the sick- this is our work. The profession in truth is a sort of guild or brotherhood, any member of which can take up his calling in any part of the world and find brethren whose language and methods and whose aims and ways are identical with his own. [9]

Find Mentors: The Young Person's Friend

Osler sought out many mentors in his life and in tribute to three of them dedicated his most celebrated book, *The Principles and Practice of Medicine,* to them. He also admired and was a serious student of many great writers, some of whose works are suggested bedside reading for all medical students so as to afford them a liberal education. Students of his day were urged to read for half an hour each day (in addition to their formal studies) from the following suggested bedside library:

Old and New Testament
Shakespeare
Montaigne
Plutarch's Lives
Marcus Aurelius
Epictetus
Religio Medici
Don Quixote
Emerson
Oliver Wendell Holmes—Breakfast-Table Series

In addition to these authors, some of Osler's historical mentors were Thomas Linacre (1450–1524), William Harvey (1578–1657), and Thomas Sydenham (1624–1689). Osler also sought opportunities to surround himself with medical students. They were frequently invited to partake in beer, biscuits, and cheese at his home on 1 West Franklin Street in Baltimore. Harvey Cushing noted, "In these surroundings he was at his best" [13]. Those particularly in his favor would be invited over 1 h earlier than the rest. Special students were also given latchkeys to his library so they could come and go as they pleased and peruse his vast collection of books. Osler looked to students to stimulate him and serve as an anecdote against premature senility. These relationships were mutually beneficial. After his death, a former student noted that he "achieved many honors and many dignities, but the proudest of all was his unwritten title, 'the Young Man's Friend'" [12].

Be Positive: "Prince of Friends and Benefactors"

Osler was by all accounts an optimist. His historical mentors Earl Nightingale, Norman Vincent Peale, and Sir Thomas Browne were all with similarly positive attitudes. In Aequanimatus, Osler urged medical students to choose their path and decide what type of doctor they were to be. He believed that we could create our own future and decide what type of life we may live. "To each one of you the practice of medicine will be very much as you make it- to one a worry, a care, a perpetual annoyance; to another, a daily joy and a life of as much happiness and usefulness as can well fall to the lot of man."

Bryan notes that "most positive people give generously, and Osler was no exception." Throughout his life he gave others what he had—be it a coat to a man shivering in the cold, tutelage to a student, or care for a patient. There are many stories of how he befriended and was of help to others. Bryan recounts one story that is especially poignant:

> Osler, on his way to an Oxford graduation and dressed in academic gown, was asked to see a small boy with severe whooping cough complicated by bronchitis. The child would not eat. The nurses and his parents tried to feed him without success. Osler did not have much time but acted as though he had plenty. He examined the child briefly and then sat down at the bedside. He carefully peeled a peach, coated it with sugar, cut it into small pieces, and offered them to the child one at a time, telling the boy that it was special fruit and that he would find it good. Hurrying off to the ceremony, he gave the boy's father a bleak prognosis: "I'm sorry Ernest but I don't think I shall see the boy again, there's very little chance when they're bad as that." Osler visited the child daily for 40 days. Because the boy had seen him as a magical figure in his academic regalia, Osler brought his robe and put it on outside the room before each visit. The child began to improve a few days after the first visit and made a full recovery.

Learn and Teach: Drive Plato's Horses

Lifelong learning was as important to Osler as was teaching. Osler, like Hippocrates, was a strong advocate that physicians sharpen their skill of observation. Observation particularly is mentioned not only by Hippocrates but Osler as well as being essential to a physician. "The whole art of medicine is in observation." Students were taught to hone not only their skills of observation but use all of their senses. A quote often attributed to Osler is "Listen to the patient, he is telling you the diagnosis."

Care Carefully: The Least Sentimental and the Most Helpful

Osler is described as someone who demonstrated care by his actions and not words. Bryan importantly notes "The physician's first duty is to be competent at what he or she professes to be able to do, and to do it consistently and well. In a sense, acts of benevolent competence are compassion, while compassion without competence is fraud." How to be competent is not the focus of this book. No matter what healing profession we are in, you will likely meet clinicians in your specialty who on the one hand are kindly, polite, warm and caring— yet their actions or clinical judgment may be grossly wrong. Likewise, you will come across others who practice state-of-the-art care. Their recommendations are evidence-based and logical. Yet their interactions with the patient are not only poor, they sabotage the relationship. A true healer in the Osler tradition would do neither. Clearly, being dedicated to lifelong learning, being observant, developing methods, and being thorough is a good start for every healer. In addition, healers must be mindful that they are taking care of a person and not a disease. If you are reading this and find yourself wanting for more, specifically an example of how you may show such compassion, I offer the following two quotes for your consideration.

First, Bryan cites a contemporary of Osler who said that his unspoken motto seemed to have been "Do the kind thing and do it first." Secondly, one of the most important lessons I believe a healer can take away from a book on the art of caring is the very practical recommendation attributed to Osler "Never leave the bedside without

a word of encouragement." Osler would likely agree with the philosophy of having unconditional positive regard for each person as promoted by the American psychologist Carl Rogers (see Chap. 8).

Additional chapters of Bryan's text explore communication skills
and the exhortation to seek balance in one's life by way of pursuing
simplicity and temperance. The reader is referred to Bryan's text for
a well-written and researched overview on the inspirational life of Sir
William Osler.

I conclude my condensed review of Osler by highlighting his success as a role model, an embodiment of the humanistic physician.
Osler understood—as did, I suspect, all of the other healers discussed
in this book—the patient's central role in the physician's work. Osler
wrote, "The good physician treats the disease; the great physician
treats the patient who has the disease." This is expanded in the notion
that "it is much more important to know what sort of patient has a
disease than what sort of disease a patient has" [5]. Osler is often
called the father of psychosomatic medicine because of his astuteness
in recognizing this key concept: when it comes to helping our patients
with their illnesses, one cannot separate the somatic from the psychological, the physical from the emotional, or the patient from his or her
unique cultural background and life experiences. One of the more
difficult challenges in the healing professions is care for the patient
with a psychosomatic illness, especially when he/she possesses little
to no insight. Often patients and their families are in denial of or hold
stigma for such illnesses, and providing your patient with proper
treatment is difficult if this is the case. In situations such as this, it
may be helpful to ease into education of the patient by telling them
of the analogy, "The body and mind are like husband and wife, when
one doesn't feel well, the other sympathizes."

In Table 4.1, Charles S. Bryan has identified ten examples of
qualities or excellences taught and modeled by William Osler that
applies to everyone[4] [6].

Sir William Osler embodied the traits of the consummate internist,
clinician, and humanistic healer. He was keenly aware of the power
of observation in caring for his patients and emphasized the importance of learning from one's personal experiences. He urged the
healer to develop an inner and outer calmness when approaching

---

[4] In his article Bryan, who also coedited *The Quotable Osler*, provides the reader
with a quote by Osler to support each admonition.

Table 4.1 Examples of qualities or excellence taught and modeled by William Osler

1.	Have ideals, preferably in writing
2.	Study time management
3.	Take care of yourself
4.	Be a positive person
5.	Take interest in your work
6.	Value education
7.	Read wisely and well
8.	Cultivate the humanities
9.	Appreciate your fellow humans
10.	Accept the human condition

difficult situations and taught that by following established methods and thorough practices, we can provide the most effective care for our patients. Osler reminds us once again that patients are more than a mix of pathologic process and disease, but they are human beings who are suffering in some physical and emotional way. He advised educating physicians in both the fields of medicine and humanities. Osler, like Hippocrates, advocated that the most successful delivery of patient care is accomplished with efforts to gain a better understanding for the *people* we strive to heal and the *artists* of medicine we wish to realize in ourselves. By looking at the life of Sir William Osler, we learn how one man strived to realize such a goal.

Francis Weld Peabody

One of the essential qualities of the clinician is interest in humanity …

–Francis Weld Peabody

Francis Weld Peabody (1881–1927) was an American medical educator (see Fig. 4.6). This distinguished physician was trained at Harvard and Johns Hopkins before returning to New England where he served as Professor of Medicine, Harvard Medical School; Director of the Thorndike Memorial Laboratory; and Visiting Physician and Chief of the Fourth Medical Service, Boston City Hospital. Like so many of the teachers chronicled in this text, his fame and memory—if known to those outside of academic medicine, may be best associated with a single quote, such as the one above. Peabody's adage to patient care appeared as an article *Care of the Patient*, which initially appeared in the Journal of the American

Fig. 4.6 Francis Weld Peabody (Courtesy of Boston Medical Center; used with permission)

Medical Association (JAMA) and later was included in a collection of Peabody's works entitled *Doctor and Patient* [14].

In *Care of the Patient*, Peabody notes that a common criticism conveyed by older practitioners is that younger graduates are over-whelmingly taught about the science of medicine, yet they lack the knowledge on how to truly *take care* of patients [14]. The early twentieth century was a time of astounding progress and discovery in the science and technology of medicine, and Peabody understood the need for teaching students of the most recent advancements. He felt that "the art of medicine and the science of medicine [were] not antagonistic but supplementary to each other," [14] a notion that was often overpowered by the common sentiment of the time that all answers could be learned through empirical experimentation and diligent analysis. Peabody noted that part of the separation of this art from science occurs because education of early twentieth century medical students occurred solely in the hospital—a sterile, technical, dehumanizing place. This concept remains valid today. All too often, hospitalized patients become identified not as who they are, but as the disease state they represent. "That case of mitral stenosis is in the second bed on the left."

Patients are worked up scientifically, represented only by specimens and samples, histological cultures, and stains, and if their extensive tests reveal an absence of physical findings or dearth of abnormal organic growth, patients may be discharged with simply, "There is nothing wrong with you." When describing inpatient medicine of his time, Peabody explained, "In hospital and in private practice ... excluding cases of acute infection, approximately half of their patients complained of symptoms for which an adequate organic cause could not be discovered" [14]. However, many patients whose work-ups yielded negative results possessed real reasons for their sicknesses. Unfortunately for them, the most recent scientific advancements of their time produced inadequate laboratory tests by today's standards and positive results were frequently missed. Of course, those patients with functional disorders constitute a group who still require treatment. It is the medical student, Peabody notes, who is given the first opportunity to speak to the newly admitted— often lonely, frightened, stripped-naked—patients upon their admission to the hospital. The student is urged to cherish this experience and use this opportunity to form a relationship with patients and to get to know them as the unique individuals they are.

After ruling out organic causes of ailment, we are urged to consider the prospect of a functional or psychosomatic disorder. The best way to reveal this is by listening to our patients. It is recommended that the young healer make sure to investigate the life events of the patient at the time of onset of his or her symptoms. Some patients lack insight into the connection between emotional and psychological experience and the physical body. The healer may have to function as a medical detective in order to bridge the gaps to diagnosis. I once saw a recent law school graduate who complained of atypical migraine-like headaches, which appeared seemingly out of nowhere. Upon further questioning, he admitted that his wife and children moved back home several states away to give him adequate space and privacy to study for the local bar exam. Although he had agreed to this arrangement, he had not anticipated the effects it would have on his happiness and physical well-being. The cause of his pain was functional and the discomfort was real. Peabody chooses patients with functional disorders to exemplify the significance of the personal relationship physicians should aim to develop with their patients, one that allows for trust between each partner and the most effective communication possible:

> The good physician knows his patients through and through, and his
> knowledge is bought dearly. Time, sympathy, and understanding must be
> lavishly dispensed, but the reward is to be found in that personal bond
> which forms the greatest satisfaction of the practice of medicine [14].

It is interesting to remind ourselves that earlier medical educators, such as Hippocrates, Rhazes, and Osler, also stressed the importance of functional illnesses and psychosomatic disorders and their impact on patient health. This is a common theme emphasized by many great practitioners throughout medicine. However, Francis Weld Peabody brought this idea to the forefront of medical practice during a time in which the scientific mindset dominated and technical experimentation and testing were valued perhaps more than less tangible, humanistic qualities. Peabody reminds us to be caring, thoughtful, and compassionate in dealing with our patients and to always remember that those we care for are people before they are patients. He ends his classic essay by noting something simple yet profound: "One of the essential qualities of the clinician is interest in humanity, for the secret of the care of the patient is in caring for the patient" [14].

Albert Schweitzer

> "I do not know your destiny, but I do know one thing: the only ones among
> you who will be really happy are those who will have sought and found
> how to serve."
>
> –Albert Schweitzer

The Alsatian Lorraine theologian, physician, philosopher, and Nobel Prize winner Albert Schweitzer (1875–1965) exemplified a life committed to serving others (see Figs. 4.7, 4.8, 4.9 and 4.10). Like Francis Weld Peabody, he was the son of a minister, born into a family that highly valued the pursuit of scholarly activities and religious study. Schweitzer received a doctorate in philosophy in 1899 and a licentiate in theology from the University of Strasbourg in 1900. By the age of 29, he was recognized as a renowned scholar in both disciplines, earning theological acclaim for his book *The Quest of the Historical Jesus*. Interestingly, Schweitzer was also an accomplished organist and earned money performing throughout Europe for much of his early life. These funds would later be utilized to establish the jungle hospital he founded in Lambaréné, now present day Gabon. He was a musicologist as well as performer

Fig. 4.7 Albert Schweitzer AS-1963-343 (Schweitzer comforts a woman who was crying because others made fun of her hunched back. Courtesy of the Albert Schweitzer Fellowship Boston, Massachusetts. All photos from: The Schweitzer Album: A portrait in words and pictures by Erica Anderson, New York Harper and Row, Publishers, 1965. Reprinted with permission: Syracuse University Library, New York)

Fig. 4.8 Albert Schweitzer AS-1963-526 (Schweitzer visiting a patient in the wards at his hospital. Courtesy of the Albert Schweitzer Fellowship Boston, Massachusetts. All photos from: The Schweitzer Album: A portrait in words and pictures by Erica Anderson, New York Harper and Row, Publishers, 1965. Reprinted with permission: Syracuse University Library, New York)

Fig. 4.9 Albert Schweitzer AS-GCN-20 (Schweitzer on the hillside near the Ogowe River at his jungle hospital during the first year. Courtesy of the Albert Schweitzer Fellowship Boston, Massachusetts. All photos from: The Schweitzer Album: A portrait in words and pictures by Erica Anderson, New York Harper and Row, Publishers, 1965. Reprinted with permission: Syracuse University Library, New York)

Fig. 4.10 Albert Schweitzer by Karsh# 1 (copyright Yousuf Karsh, karsh.org)
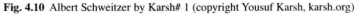

and published a biography of Johan Sebastian Bach in French in 1905, a book on organ building and playing in 1906, and rewrote the Bach book in German in 1908. Schweitzer recognized that he was born to privilege and when he was only 21 made the decision that upon turning 30, he would dedicate his life to the service of others.

Having determined to go to Africa as a medical missionary rather than as a pastor, Schweitzer began the study of medicine at the University of Strasbourg in 1905. After obtaining his MD degree in 1913, he founded the hospital that now bears his name at Lambaréné in French Equatorial Africa. In 1917, Schweitzer and his wife were sent to a French internment camp as prisoners of war. Released in 1918, Schweitzer returned to Europe and spent the next 6 years preaching in his old church, giving lectures and concerts, taking medical courses, and writing. Schweitzer published many texts including: *The Decay and Restoration of Civilization* (1923), *Christianity and the Religions of the World* (1923), *On the Edge of the Primeval Forest* (1931), and *Civilization and Ethics* (1946). Like several of the healers we discuss in this book, Schweitzer was an advocate for ethical behavior and service to those less fortunate. On these humanistic notions, Schweitzer writes to a group of nursing students:

> You ask me to give you a motto. Here it is: service. Let this word accompany you as you seek your way and your duty in the world. May it be recalled to your minds if ever you are tempted to forget it or to set it aside. Never have this word on your lips, but keep it in your hearts. And may it be a confidant that will teach you not only to do good but to do it simply and humbly. It will not always be a comfortable companion but it will always be a faithful one. And it will be able to lead you to happiness, no matter what the experiences of your lives are [15].

Marvin Meyer, the Director of the Albert Schweitzer Institute at Chapman University, writes in his forward for *Reverence for Life: The Ethics of Albert Schweitzer for the Twenty-First Century* that Schweitzer preached how "all of us are brothers and sisters of the suffering; we all belong to each other" [16]. Schweitzer taught that we no longer belong to ourselves and that we must help those suffering, calling this the "fellowship of those who bear the mark of pain." This concept remains true today. As healthcare professionals, we are directly involved with those who suffer. We are ourselves privileged to fulfill this role yet are also affected in some way by each healthcare interaction we experience. Every patient leaves an impression—a mark—and by taking what is important from those we provide care to, we may learn and grow as physicians. It may often seem that we belong to our patients, especially in a society in which we are sought out for specific skills, paid for service, and judged by both objective and subjective standards. However, our patients provide us service as well: the chance to learn from them, to improve our own abilities, and to provide better care in the future.

In addition to living a life of compassion and service, Schweitzer was known for his philosophy of the "reverence for life," which he considered to be his greatest contribution to mankind. His daughter, Rhena Schweitzer Miller is quoted as reflecting upon a conversation she had with her father one day, in which she asked him, "You have done so much for Africa. Has it given you anything in return?" He said, "Yes, nowhere else could I have found the idea of reverence for life than here" [16]. The story of how Schweitzer came upon this concept is quite interesting. In his book *Out of My Life and Thought*, Schweitzer describes how he made the conscious decision to reflect upon his personal values and understandings of the world. While taking a trip on the Ogowe River, he put to words the core notions of his philosophical thought. Below is a passage that describes how he came to this revelation:

> Slowly we crept upstream, laboriously navigating—it was the dry season between the sandbanks. Lost in thought I sat on the deck of the barge, struggling to find the elementary and universal concept of the ethical that I had not discovered in any philosophy. I covered sheet after sheet with disconnected sentences merely to concentrate on the problem. Two days passed. Late on the third day, at the very moment when, at sunset, we were making our way through a herd of hippopotamuses, there flashed upon my mind, unforeseen and unsought, the phrase 'reverence for life.' The iron door had yielded. The path in the thicket had become visible. Now I had found my way to the principle in which affirmation of the world and ethics are joined together! [17]

We learn by looking at the life of Albert Schweitzer that his role as a great healer was only a part of his legendary history. He contributed as a philosopher, pastor, theologian, musician, and a prominent social activist. Schweitzer served not only people who were suffering—one patient at a time—but also mankind, as he made significant attempts to improve social health as a whole. For example, Schweitzer put forth extensive effort to immediately end atmospheric nuclear test explosions. Through careful analysis, ongoing and convincing presentation, he showed the harmful effects of radioactive fallout on humankind and the environment, and he continued working to abolish the use of nuclear weapons completely. Schweitzer was given the Nobel Peace Prize in 1952, although it was withheld until December

10, 1953. Because of hospital duties, he was unable to come to Oslo to claim the award until 1954. His Nobel Prize speech entitled, "The Problem of Peace" [18] is considered by some to be one of the greatest speeches ever given. Part of this speech extols wealthier nations to be responsible for other nations, which were not as fortunate. "What really matters is that we should all of us realize that we are guilty of inhumanity" [16]. With the $33,000 prize money, he completed construction of the leprosarium at Lambaréné, a new facility considered so state-of-the-art that Schweitzer once said, "Now everyone is going to want to have leprosy!" [15]

Albert Schweitzer died on September 4, 1965 and was buried at Lambaréné. He strongly supported the notion that an individual's life and practices should match his or her beliefs. "A man's life should be the same as his thought." Of himself, Schweitzer confirmed, "I have made my life my argument" [15]. Perhaps the greatest lesson that healers of any age can learn from Albert Schweitzer is that we possess the potential to put our beliefs into action and that in doing so—by living in accordance with our own ideals—we may find the deepest satisfaction possible. From a practical standpoint, few, if any, of us may feel capable of leaving our current reality to travel halfway around the world and commit ourselves to our work and people in a way similar to Schweitzer. This great man found solace in commitment toward helping humankind. Although many may not fathom his decisions—that is, practicing in a primeval forest hospital in war-torn third world countries—he teaches us that accomplishments in medicine are subjective in their effect on society and the single physician. Further, that each member of health care may find true fulfillment in their medical practice and life's work. May "everyone have his (or her) own Lambaréné."

References

1. Mosby CV. A little journey to the home of Florence Nightingale. St. Louis, MO: The Press of CV Mosby Company; 1938.
2. Dossey B, Selanders L, Beck D, Attewell A. Florence Nightingale today: healing leadership global action. Silver Spring, MD: American Nurses Association; 2005.
3. Nightingale F. Notes on nursing and hospitals. Birmingham AL: The Classics of Medicine Library; 1982.
4. Pennock MR. Makers of nursing history. New York: Lakeside Publishing Company; 1940.

5. Mackowiak P. Post mortem: solving histories great medical mysteries. Philadelphia, PA: American College of Physicians; 2007.
6. Osler, W. Aequanimatus, McGraw-Hill, Third Edition, The Blakiston Division, New York, 1 Mar 1989.
7. Osler Library Newsletter, no. 108, 2007 Osler Library of the History of Medicine. McGill University, Montréal (Québec) Canada. http://en.wikipedia.org/wiki/William_Osler. Accessed May 2009. http://www.mcgill.ca/files/osler-library/No1082007.pdf
8. Osler, W. Preface to the second edition: Oxford July 1906. Aequanimatus, 3rd ed. New York: McGraw-Hill, Inc.; 1939
9. Osler, W. Teacher and student. Valedictory address to University of Minnesota, 1892. Aequanimatus. 3rd ed. New York: McGraw-Hill, Inc.; 1939. p. 23–41
10. Institute of Medicine. Committee on Quality of Health Care in America. To err is human: building a safer health system. Washington, DC: National Academy Press; 2000.
11. Bryan CS. Osler: inspirations from a great physician. 1st ed. New York: Oxford University Press; 1997.
12. Bryan CS. What is the oslerian tradition. Ann Intern Med. 1994;1(20):8.
13. Cushing H. The life of Sir William Osler. Oxford: Clarendon; 1925.
14. Peabody FW. Doctor and patient. New York: The Macmillan Company; 1930.
15. http://www.schweitzerfellowship.org/features/about/phil/
16. Meyer M. Reverence for Life: The Ethics of Albert Schweitzer for the Twenty-First Century Edited By: Marvin Meyer and Kurt BergelReviewed Edition: Syracuse University Press, Syracuse, New York, 2002ISBN 0-8156-2977-XSoftcover, 350 pages. Reference accesible by goint to: http://home.pcisys.net/~jnf/schabout/ra20.html
17. Schweitzer A. Out of my life and thought: an autobiography. New York/Baltimore, MD: Henry Holte and Co./Johns Hopkins University Press; 1998. Trans. Antje Bultmann Lemke.
18. Schweitzer A (1954) The problem of peace. Nobel lecture http://nobelprize.org/nobel_prizes/peace/laureates/1952/schweitzer-lecture.html

Nightingale

Nightingale F. Notes on nursing and hospitals. Birmingham, AL: The Classics of Medicine Library; 1982.

Osler

The Osler history of medicine library at McGill University houses a tremendous number of resources, references, photos, and other links related to the works of Sir William Osler. http://www.mcgill.ca/osler-library
References cited by Osler History of Medicine Library include

Bliss M. William Osler: a life in medicine. Toronto, ON: University of Toronto Press; 1999.

Bryan CS. What is the oslerian tradition. Ann Intern Med. 1994;1(20):8.

Cushing H. The life of Sir William Osler. Oxford: Clarendon; 1925.

Osler SW. Aphorisms from his bedside teachings and writings. 2nd ed. Springfield, IL: Thomas Publishers; 1961.

Osler W. The Quotable Osler – Revised Paperback Edition [Kindle Edition], Mark E. Silverman (Author, Editor), Charles S. Bryan (Author, Editor), T. Jock Murray (Editor) File Size: 1048 KB, Print Length: 318 pages Publisher: American College of Physicians (September 1, 2007) Sold by: Amazon Digital Services

Osler W. Obituaries: Sir William Osler. Br Med J. 1920;1:30.

Bryan CS. Osler inspirations from a great physician. New York: Oxford University Press; 1977.

Additional WWW sites with material by or about Sir William Osler, as suggested by The Osler Library of the History of Medicine are

Ask Osleriana—A Searchable Database of Osler Essays

Celebrating the contributions of William Osler, 1849–1919, an online collection of photographs, writings and letters of Sir William Osler created by the Alan Mason Chesney Medical Archives of the Johns Hopkins Medical Institution (JHMI)

Visitors to Baltimore should visit the Welch Library at JHMI and view the large painting of "The Four Greats" hanging in the second floor reading room, depicting the images of Osler, Halstead, Welch and Kelly. Across the street from this library, at Johns Hopkins Hospital, you may also make a reservation to view the Osler room, where he wrote The principles and practice of medicine and which houses memorabilia that may interest those interested in the life of Sir William Osler

The American Osler Society was founded for the purpose of bringing together members of the medical and allied professions who are, by their common inspiration, dedicated to memorialize and perpetuate the just and charitable life, the intellectual resourcefulness, and the ethical example of Sir William Osler (1849–1919). http://www.americanosler.org/

Schweitzer

Schweitzer A. Out of my life and thought: an autobiography. New York/ Baltimore, MD: Henry Holte and Co./Johns Hopkins University Press; 1998. Trans. Antje Bultmann Lemke.

Schweitzer A. Essential writings. Maryknoll, New York: Orbis Books; 2005. Sel. James Brazabon.

The Albert Schweitzer Institute

The Albert Schweitzer Institute of Chapman University is dedicated to the task of preserving, critically interpreting, and disseminating the ethical teachings of Albert Schweitzer within the context of the study of ethics and ethical values. The Institute sponsors a university course on the life and thought of Albert Schweitzer, maintains an Albert Schweitzer Exhibit on the campus of Chapman University, offers the Albert Schweitzer Award of Excellence and Schweitzer scholarships, and participates in academic programs on the legacy of Albert Schweitzer. Their website has useful and interesting information for those wanting to learn more about the life of Albert Schweitzer, and can be accessed at www.chapman.edu/SchweitzerInstitute

Another university-based website that is useful to learn more about the life of Albert Schweitzer is housed at Quinnipiac University and is accessible by visiting www.quinnipiac.edu

Albert Schweitzer Nobel prize acceptance speech, "The Problem with Peace" can be read in its entirety by visiting http://nobelprize.org/nobel_prizes/peace/laureates/1952/schweitzer-lecture.html

The Albert Schweitzer Fellowship sends third-year medical students to spend 3 months working as Fellows at the Albert Schweitzer Hospital in Lambaréné, Gabon, on clinical rotations. The mission of the Albert Schweitzer Fellowship is to develop "leaders in service." These are individuals who are dedicated and skilled in addressing the health needs of underserved communities and whose example influences and inspires others. More information can be obtained at http://www.Schweitzerfellowship.org

Schweitzer A. On the edge of the primeval forest (Zwischen Wasser und Urwald). London/New York: A. & C. Black/Holt Rinehart and Winston; 1958. Trans. C.T. Campion.

Schweitzer A. My life and thought. London/New York: George Allen and Unwin/Henry Holt; 1993/1948. Trans. C.T. Campion.

Chapter 5
Modern Masters

Theodore E. Woodward

Our noble profession would be well served if the public could be made aware of its more human side.

–Theodore E. Woodward

Our next great teacher served at an institution very close to my heart, the University of Maryland School of Medicine. Theodore E. Woodward (1914–2005) is one of the most notable physicians to hold the position of Chairman of Medicine (see Fig. 5.1). Dr. Woodward received his M.D. degree from the University of Maryland School of Medicine in 1938 and became a nationally and internationally renowned authority in infectious diseases. He was instrumental in reporting the first cure for typhus and typhoid fever during World War II, which earned him a nomination for a Nobel Prize in Medicine in 1948. Dr. Woodward was acknowledged by his alma mater for undeniable dedication to teaching and commitment to patients. Over the years he received many awards, some of which include the Golden Apple Teaching Award from the University of Maryland (over a dozen times) and the Faculty Award for outstanding abilities as a teacher (over 20 times). He was a founding father of the field of infectious diseases and globally acknowledged as the premier expert on Rickettsial diseases. The details of Dr. Woodward's numerous accomplishments are not appropriate for this text, but his impact on world heath was and continues to be profound.

R. Colgan, *Advice to the Healer: On the Art of Caring*,
DOI 10.1007/978-1-4614-5170-9_5,
© Springer Science+Business Media, LLC 2013

Fig. 5.1 (**a**) Theodore Woodward (Laughing, Courtesy of Medical Alumni Association of the University of Maryland, Inc.; used with permission). (**b**) Theodore Woodward (In front of Microscope, Courtesy of Medical Alumni Association of the University of Maryland, Inc.; used with permission)

Aside from his great accomplishments as researcher, academician, and trailblazer in infectious disease, I have included Woodward in this book because of his contributions to the art of medicine and how he exemplified excellence by the life he chose to live. While some academic physicians climb over others to get to higher professional levels, Woodward was famous for helping others fulfill their potential. According to his longtime friend and colleague, Dr. Philip A. Mackowiak, he was also generous to a fault—aiding others in their careers and research at the expense of his own accomplishments.

Dr. Mackowiak, the Chief of Medicine at the Baltimore Veterans Administration Medical Center, was himself a mentee of Dr. Woodward. Modeling his life and practice after his mentor, Mackowiak is also known by his students for his clinical astuteness, kindness, and care of the patient. Dr. Mackowiak cites a long list of physicians taught by Woodward who went on to high positions of leadership. In the foreword to Woodward's book *Make Room for Sentiment*, Dr. Mackowiak notes, "He will long be remembered in the minds of physicians, here and abroad, not for what he has received but for what he has contributed" [1].

Woodward had an incredible work ethic and sense of duty to his patients. Dr. Mackowiak regularly illustrates this point to the many students rotating through the Baltimore VAMC with a story of his mentor's dedication. A prime example of this extraordinary dedication occurred 1 day during a Baltimore blizzard. Dr. Mackowiak recounts that as chief of medicine, he felt it his duty to venture into the hospital on this particularly snowy day. He suspected that there would likely not be too much to attend to, but (just to be sure) he made his rounds as normal. This exhausting task took much longer than expected, and at the end of the day Dr. Mackowiak found himself collapsing into his chair, "head in (his) hands wondering how (he) would get home." As he looked up—much to his surprise—he saw Dr. Woodward standing in the door frame. His mentor (at the time in his 80s) stood in front of him in galoshes, a fur cap, and an old army jacket covered in snow and ice. It had long been known that Dr. Woodward no longer had any direct patient care responsibilities. Dr. Mackowiak inquired how it was that he arrived at the hospital. What was the purpose? Frankly, "Why are you here?" To which Dr. Woodward replied: "I hitched a ride on a snow plow." (Personal communication) This story exemplifies the sense of duty and professionalism by which Dr. Woodward lived. This is just one example of many that illustrates this man's commitment to his profession and his patients and is one of the many reasons Dr. Woodward is regarded by Dr. Mackowiak as "my hero."

Dr. Woodward was known for his great sense of humor and his practical approach to clinical diagnosis. He would often spend over an hour with new patients, getting to know every detail of their life story. One caution he often passed on to medical students was the warning: "Don't be a slip doctor." A "slip" is the shortened way of referring to the "lab slip," the paper form students and house staff filled out in the pre-computer age. Dr. Woodward felt that we should sit down and talk to our patients and come to a clinical diagnosis based upon a careful analysis of the history and physical and not rely solely upon ordering laboratory tests. Dr. Woodward's most popular proverb is recognized around the country and perhaps the world. The saying is:

> If you are walking down Greene Street (the street in front of University Hospital in Baltimore) and you hear hoof beats behind you, don't look back expecting to see a zebra. Expect a horse.

In other words: common things occur commonly.

Theodore Woodward had time for anyone wanting to learn. Alas, the only personal contact I had with Dr. Woodward was when I sought his help in creating a bioterrorism presentation. I was invited by Dr. Woodward to look through his slide carousel for any slides I might like to use for my talk. In this deck were photos he had taken during his decades of work, including documentation of those with typhus, cholera, and assorted infectious diseases. When I was invited to sit down with him in his cluttered office down the hall from Dr. Mackowiak at the Baltimore VAMC, I knew that I shared company of one of the greatest physicians of our century. Dr. Woodward was careful and cautious even in his later years. True to protocol and procedure, when I offered to have all of his slides converted into digital media he turned me down, saying simply, "No, it will get out of hand."

And like so many of the great teachers reviewed thus far, Woodward shares—besides, of course, his accomplishments as a clinician, leader, guardian of the public's health, and educator—his belief in service. In one of the many addresses he gave to the graduating students at the University of Maryland School of Medicine, Woodward made the following remarks to the class of 1983:

> Our noble profession would be well served if the public could be made aware of its more human side. A home visit or even a telephone call after a patient has been informed that he has cancer, being present during the time of dying or in the operating room when surgery is performed or attending a former patient's funeral serve those purposes well. Acceptance of these responsibilities and the discharging of them are the characteristics of a complete physician. —[Personal communication (copy of speech transcript) Phillip Mackowiak]

Even a few years before his death at the age of 91, Theodore Woodward could still be seen walking slowly down the halls of University Hospital with his black bag in hand and a group of second-year medical students by his side.

Edmund D. Pellegrino

> Do good and avoid evil is the primum principium of all ethics.
>
> –Edmund D. Pellegrino

One of America's greatest physician-educators in the areas of professional ethics and bioethics is Edmund D. Pellegrino

Fig. 5.2 Edmund Pellegrino (Courtesy of the American Medical Association, as supplied by the President's Council on Bioethics; used with permission)

(see Fig. 5.2). Dr. Pellegrino has been Professor Emeritus of Medicine and Medical Ethics at the Center for Clinical Bioethics at Georgetown University Medical Center since 2001. In 2004, he was named to the International Bioethics Committee of the United Nations Educational and Scientific and Cultural Organization, and in 2005 he became the chairman of the President's Council on Bioethics. Dr. Pellegrino is a prolific author and founding editor of the *Journal of Medicine and Philosophy*.

While bioethics and the philosophy of medicine may be viewed as a theoretical dilemma perhaps too overwhelming and time-consuming for the busy practitioner, the Pellegrino reader comes to understand that recognition of such profound notions is as important as taking patients' vital signs. Indeed Dr. Pellegrino makes a convincing argument that the philosophy of medicine, bioethics, and the physician–patient relationship cannot be separated from one another, and in fact these exist in a very complex and entwined relationship. In interviewing Dr. Pellegrino for this book, I was at first surprised when he asked *me* to define what *I* meant by the term "the art of medicine," reminding me that this concept may mean different things to different people. He pointed out that the area which I seemed to be most interested in might best be described in the context of the physician–patient relationship.[1] Dr. Pellegrino took great effort to remind me that it is this moral bond between a healer and his patient that must be cherished and safeguarded.

Many of the works of Pellegrino may prove difficult to interpret for the nonphilosopher or those not fully accustomed to academic jargon. I know that I lack the educational background and knowledge base to bring the ideas of some of the great philosophers together in a manner as eloquently as he does in creating a cogent argument for his positions. Yet I immediately sat upright when I heard him speak of the "non-philosopher philosopher." I thought—that's me (and likely you). And truly this is another fantastic aspect of our combined vocations, the fact that we are allowed to be intimate with the human condition and invited into the lives of others. Once within this inner sanctum we are privy to things that no one else may ever know or learn. This gives every clinician pause and an opportunity to speculate and admire. I believe all healers are more or less "non-philosopher philosophers," because at a minimum we *wonder*. And, according to Plato, Socrates cites in Theaetetus "all philosophy begins with wonder" [2].

It is an obvious injustice and impossibility to distill the entirety of Dr. Pellegrino's works into a few pages, and I won't. Yet if we seriously want to try to understand how to be the best healers we can, we must recognize that a significant aspect of the physician–patient relationship involves medical ethics. Dr. Pellegrino explains, "The first principle of medical ethics, the end to which it is directed, is the good of the patient." This principle can be traced back to the time of Hippocrates:

> I will follow that system or regimen, which according to my ability and judgment I consider for the benefit of my patient and abstain from whatever is deleterious and mischievous [3].

In his essay *The Commodification of Medical and Health Care* [4] Dr. Pellegrino begins with a passage from *Book I* of *The Republic*, in which Socrates asks Thrasymachus this question:

> But tell me, your physician in the precise sense of whom you were just speaking, is he a moneymaker, an earner of fees or a healer of the sick? [5]

---

[1] In the pages to follow, I take the liberty of expanding on Dr. Pellegrino's thoughts to suggest that when he speaks of the physician I believe it to be relevant to nonphysician clinicians as well.

Dr. Pellegrino applies this notion to modern times, that today many people view our profession as having undergone a paradigm shift from a profession to a business entity. It is important to distinguish this misconception. The technician, who has learned the trade, is a member of the business community of medicine. The healer, who always keeps the patient as the center of his focus "knows the art." Physicians are often challenged to choose what is best for the patient versus what is best for the corporate bottom line. Pellegrino notes that health care cannot be a commodity, given the special nature of illness and healing [4]. We in the healing professions are afforded a special privilege by society, one that begins with the permission to learn from cadavers and extends upwards to the clinical years as we gain rudimentary skills on willing patients. Because of this special privilege, Dr. Pellegrino rightfully recognizes that we have tacitly entered into a contract with society to use the knowledge we acquire from these allowances for the benefit of those who are sick. We are urged to refrain from substituting the word "consumers" for patients or "providers" for doctors. We are urged to remain physicians and to be concerned with healing and not moneymaking.

There exist many instances where physicians are seduced to make more money by doing things for the patient which may be unnecessary. An example that came to my attention was an ambulatory medical group that hires physicians for a base salary. The physician's income is potentially increased by incentive bonuses, paid out to the contractor based in part on the number of additional dollars earned through ordering in-house ancillary services and tests. This type of activity can easily be seen as encouraging, even promoting, a potential conflict of interest between what is best for the patient and what is best for the moneymaking physician. The physician achieves his or her bonus by ordering increased number of tests, but it is the patient who is subjected to these unnecessary tests and possibly invasive procedures. This situation just doesn't pass the sniff test: If something smells bad, perhaps it is bad.

Pellegrino feels that healers should not be gatekeepers or rationers of health care, but of course we cannot prevent this by ourselves. Society must ensure that health care does not become a commodity, and the most effective means to accomplish this is through policy, politics, and regulations. We, as physicians, possess the obligation to show them why they should put forth the effort to strive for this health care ideal. For society to take on this quest, we must convince our patients that we hold the faith in our profession as something sacred.

If health care is for sale then the physician is indeed a moneymaker. Pellegrino ends his discussion on medicine as a commodity with another quote by Plato, suggesting the ethical path for all physicians, namely,

> Can we deny, then, said I, that neither does any physician, insofar as he is a physician, seek to enjoin the advantage of the physician but that of the patient? [6]

If by reading this book your aspiration is to be best healer you can be, then as a philosopher of medicine, medical ethicist, and clinician-educator, Dr. Pellegrino will tell you that you must also recognize your role as a moral agent. On a regular basis healers must contend with certain morally questionable practices and determine how they will respond. Some specific examples include refusal to work with those who are HIV positive for fear of contagion, denying service to the poor or those with little or no insurance, cooperating with hospital authorities in discharging patients earlier than you think is reasonable, and marketing to increase the demand of dubious procedures, tests, or supplements. Pellegrino adds:

> To me the most important thing in a relationship is that the heart of the relationship is a moral enterprise that occurs between not only the doctor and his patient but the lawyer and his client, the minister and his confessor, and the teacher and his student. All of these relationships have a dependent person who needs help, who goes to another person who professes to be able to help. They enter into a fiduciary relationship (Personal Communication July 2008)

We are urged to be virtuous. Plato listed four cardinal virtues: fortitude, temperance, justice, and wisdom. Dr. Pellegrino, in writing of the virtues in medical practice, has extended this list to include fidelity to trust, compassion, integrity, self-effacement, and "phronesis." Phronesis is a term used by Aristotle to denote practical wisdom or the capacity for moral insight [7]. It seems reasonable that healers should strive to attain these virtues. In discussing virtue within the context of practicing medicine, Dr Pellegrino writes that virtue is aligned with excellence in living the good life:

> This excellence depends upon knowledge of good, evil, and self. It is not specialized knowledge directed to any one activity but rather to living one's whole life well. It must, like an art, be perfected through practice [8].

The virtuous physician must also be a virtuous person. This physician has character traits that define him as such and can be seen following his life according to a moral law. The virtuous physician is someone we can trust to do the right thing and to act courageously, honestly, justly, wisely, and temperately, according to Pellegrino. The virtuous physician will act well and with decent moral code even when others are not watching. While not defining the virtuous physician in specific detail, Dr. Pellegrino gives us some hints as to how he or she may be recognized. The virtuous physician is:

1. A person of character—someone who can be predictably trusted to act well in most circumstances and who does not yield to the allures of power, pleasure, or self-interest.
2. Someone who follows the internal morality of the (medical) profession. Profession is defined by Dr. Pellegrino as "a declaration of a way of life that is specific, a way of life in which expert knowledge is used not primarily for personal gain but for the benefit of those who need that knowledge" [8].
3. Someone who practices altruistic beneficence, which implies "not only taking the interests of others into account but doing so in such fashion that our intentions and acts give some degree of preference to the intentions of others" [8].

Outwardly, the virtuous clinician acting as an appropriate moral agent will exhibit behaviors characterized by fidelity to trust and promise, benevolence, effacement of self-interest, compassion and caring, intellectual honesty, justice, and prudence. Pellegrino also indicates that the virtuous physician is one who is consistent and acts morally both at work and at home, both in professional and personal arenas, with colleagues and patients, as well as family and friends. The physician's behaviors are not just seen while he or she is practicing medicine, but in all of his or her actions in all sections of life. Unfortunately, discrepancies occur and may negatively affect one realm as expense for maintaining another. An example of such a discrepancy is the physician who is "married" to work and doesn't have time for his or her spouse or children. A key condition of being virtuous is balancing conflicting obligations judiciously. The virtuous physician is one who acts with the "right reason," which Aristotle and Aquinas considered essential [7]. He or she realizes that one may easily be pulled in many directions by all different facets of life, but through thoughtful judgment is able to balance these opposing forces in order to achieve success in all areas. Clearly, in order to be a great healer, one must also strive to be a *virtuous* healer.

When I asked which of his many scholarly publications he considered most effective in communicating the importance of the physician–patient relationship to the young healer, who strives to be the best he or she can be with regard to the art of medicine, Dr. Pellegrino quickly cited *A Philosophical Reconstruction of Medical Morality and the Caring Ethic* [9].

In his publication, Pellegrino first describes how there exists a philosophical foundation for the obligations which bind those who profess to practice medicine, "better still, all who profess to heal" [9]. He notes that today fewer physicians follow a religious foundation of ethics or remain faithful to the Hippocratic Oath.[2]

Pellegrino proposes a philosophy of the physician–patient relationship beginning with the tenet that the physician is in all aspects of life a good man or woman. Second, he explains that the nature of medicine itself is a profession—a vocation—based on healing; further, that this raises certain expectations and implies particular requirements on the part of the physician. In this essay, Pellegrino discusses Scribonius Largus, who practiced as either a physician or pharmacist—we do not know which—in the time of the Emperor Claudius. He was one of the first to refer to medicine as a vocation in the first century ACE [10]. Scribonius opined that physicians should choose to play the role required of their profession and strive to achieve the expectations implied by their position. Commiseration and humaneness are cited as unique virtues of our profession, just as truth is to a judge.

The third source of a professional basis of ethics is the physician–patient relationship itself. Throughout medical history, physicians evolved from serving as craftsman in the time of the early Greeks to being members of an elite group in society from whom patients sought care. At one point in time, physicians directed their patients like children, educated them in how to behave or care for themselves, in a true paternalistic manner. Pellegrino notes:

> Most Greek physicians in Hippocrates time were money grubbers … While at the same time there were also physicians for freemen who provided information to their patients and gave them choices. By taking the Hippocratic Oath physicians made their commitment to indicate publically

---

[2] The reader will note that many of those highlighted in this book in fact have been identified as leaders in each of their respective religious groups.

that they were not the run of the mill practitioners … This same motive
was a factor in the 1847 Oath of the American Medical Association
(Personal communication July 2008)

Subsequent Jewish, Christian, and Islamic religious influences, in
which the self-worth of every human being is emphasized, have led
to the evolution of medicine as we know it today. Contemporary
medicine is based on the development of the physician–patient relationship as a team, a partnership in which both members make decisions about the patient's individualized health care plan. Furthermore,
Pellegrino argues that what the physician professes and the patient
expects is a right and good healing process that is specific for each
patient and his or her unique illnesses. Implicit in this "right and good
healing process" is that the physician will be technically competent.
In addition, the virtuous physician is one who ensures a moral bond
with patients by providing the information necessary for the patients
to make an informed decision about their care, while at the same time
showing respect and consideration for the patients' wishes. If the
patients cannot be their own advocate, then we must look to their
surrogate (their family, guardian, or the courts) for guidance, while
being as sure as possible that they do in fact have the patient's best
interests at heart.

The American Medical Association (AMA) has a long history of
recognizing the ethical basis of medical practice and identifies
responsibility to the patient as foremost [11]. The *Principles of
Medical Ethics* noted below are not laws, but standards of conduct
adopted by the AMA's House of Delegates on June 17, 2001.

Principles of Medical Ethics

- A physician shall be dedicated to providing competent medical
  care, with compassion and respect for human dignity and rights.
- A physician shall uphold the standards of professionalism, be honest in all professional interactions, and strive to report physicians
  deficient in character or competence, or engaging in fraud or
  deception, to appropriate entities.
- A physician shall respect the law and also recognize a responsibility to seek changes in those requirements which are contrary to the
  best interests of the patient.

- A physician shall respect the rights of patients, colleagues, and other health professionals, and shall safeguard patient confidences and privacy within the constraints of the law.
- A physician shall continue to study, apply, and advance scientific knowledge, maintain a commitment to medical education, make relevant information available to patients, colleagues, and the public, obtain consultation, and use the talents of other health professionals when indicated.
- A physician shall, in the provision of appropriate patient care, except in emergencies, be free to choose whom to serve, with whom to associate, and the environment in which to provide medical care.
- A physician shall recognize a responsibility to participate in activities contributing to the improvement of the community and the betterment of public health.
- A physician shall, while caring for a patient, regard responsibility to the patient as paramount.
- A physician shall support access to medical care for all people.

In the *Caring Ethic*, Pellegrino further explores the evolution of the physician–patient relationship. With the introduction of scientific means of therapeutics, *curing* is indeed more prevalent, yet the *caring* aspect of health care is exceedingly neglected. The concept of care can be understood within the context of the physician–patient relationship in four ways: (1) compassion, (2) doing for others what they cannot do for themselves, (3) taking care of the medical problem, and lastly (4) "taking care" to accomplish the necessary medical protocol with conscientious attention to detail. Each physician has a moral obligation to his or her patient, and Pellegrino argues for the integration of these four elements into a unified notion of care. The following anecdote speaks to this concept.

Frank M. Calia, M.D., MACP, is Professor Emeritus and former Chair of Medicine and Vice Dean for Clinical Affairs at the University Of Maryland School Of Medicine. He is a true leader in medical education, and I was fortunate to be in the audience when he spoke to an entering class of medical students on their first day of matriculation to medical school. Dr. Calia told these new medical students that in medicine there will come times when you are not sure what to do, how to proceed, or what should be done next. He then advised them to remember four simple words: "Focus on the patient." His advice reminded me of what I could imagine Hippocrates, Maimonides,

Peabody, Nightingale or Osler might have said as they instructed their apprentices. He further explained if you never forget to focus on the patient, everything else will fall in proper order. This parallels Peabody's sentiment that "the secret in the care of the patient is in caring for the patient" and mirrors Pellegrino's argument for a *unified notion of care*.

Pellegrino closes with a discussion defining humanistic character-istics of the medical profession. As physicians, when we are sought out to help our patients, we are professing to be competent and more-over that we will strive to use this competency to improve their total health, in all aspects of social, emotional, and physiological life. This is "a promise that we will not place our own interest first, that we will not exploit the vulnerability of those we serve, that we will honor the trust that illness forces upon those who are ill" [9]. Dr. Pellegrino challenges the professed healer, the "one who declares aloud" to be mindful of and faithful to the fact that this role dictates a moral responsibility to uphold ethics in the practice of his or her art. He reminds us that the profession of medicine has its own unique phi-losophy which unites those who are called to this vocation, and more-over that these accepted medical ethics are based upon the unique relationship between the physician and patient.

I am grateful for Dr. Pellegrino's encouragement to complete this book. "Books like yours stopped 30 years ago," he told me bluntly, and this strengthened my enthusiasm as I realized he—this amazing, caring, and dedicated role model of a physician—shared my feelings for its necessity. At the end of our meeting, I was taken aback as he bid me farewell. "Be good," he whispered as we shook hands in the doorway of his office at the President's Council on Bioethics in Washington, D.C. Truly, a genuine and fitting piece of advice to come from one of the most important medical philosophers of our time.

Paul Farmer

Everyone has the right to a standard of living adequate for the health and well-being of himself and of his family, including food, clothing, housing and medical care and necessary social services, and the right to security in the event of unemployment, sickness, disability, widowhood, old age, or other lack of livelihood in circumstances beyond his control.

–Universal Declaration of Human Rights, Article 25

Fig. 5.3 Paul Farmer (Courtesy of Gilles Peress, as supplied by Partners in Health/Harvard Medical School, Boston, MA; used with permission)

> I argue that equity is the central challenge for the future of medicine and public health.
>
> –Paul Farmer

Paul Farmer (1959–) is a physician, medical-anthropologist, and health advocate who strongly believes the biggest challenge facing medicine in the twenty-first century is "harnessing science to help the sick and the destitute sick" [12]. Farmer holds the positions of the Presley Professor of Medical Anthropology at Harvard Medical School and Chief of the Division of Social Medicine and Health Inequalities at Boston's Brigham and Women's Hospital (see Fig. 5.3). He is a founding director of Partners in Health, an international charity organization that provides direct health care services and advocates on behalf of the sick and poor. Farmer is also medical director of a charity hospital, the Clinique Bon Sauveur, in rural Haiti. His life story was superbly written and introduced to the public in *Mountains Beyond Mountains* by Pulitzer Prize winner Tracy Kidder. Farmer is the winner of the MacArthur Foundation Genius Award and of the Margaret Mead Award for his contributions to public anthropology. He exemplifies an expert mastery of the art of caring which is worthy of emulation. Dr. Farmer was chosen for inclusion in this book because of the personal sacrifices he has made to serve the poor, as well as his efforts in educating others about the inequalities in housing, nutrition, and health care inflicted on the destitute poor by those in power. His attention to the inequality of health care to the most vulnerable members of our society and his efforts to alleviate this disparity are nothing less than admirable.

In my mind, practicing excellence in the art of caring by attempting to master the clinician–patient relationship evokes an image of a one-to-one interaction between the healer and his or her patient. Farmer's love and concern for his individual patients is detailed beautifully in Kidder's book, including the care he has provided not only to the poor in Haiti over the past 20 years but also to those in the Soviet Union, South America, and elsewhere. This mentor gained his fame not by seeking it, but by purely promoting a better way of providing health to an underserved subsection of society—those who are without the basic necessities assumed, even expected, to be available in many parts of the world. Farmer argues that "anyone who wishes to be considered humane has ample cause to consider what it means to be sick and poor in the era of globalization and scientific advancement" [12]. This is in stark contrast to those who must suffer through illness in areas of the world without access to appropriate care or those willing to help. We are given many examples to consider in any one of his several books (see additional reading below).

Farmer's *Pathologies of Power: Health, Human Rights, and the New War on the Poor* won the 2006 J.I. Staley Prize for outstanding work in anthropology. In his text, the physician–anthropologist reveals that the most basic of human rights—the right to survive—is being denied to the most vulnerable of our world's population. Freedom from want is the human right most applicable, and unfortunately most denied to many of his patients. Physicians, nurses, and physician assistants of course need access to medicines and supplies to physically practice medicine and nursing, yet he challenges us to be more active in social and economic rights as a logical extension of care of the patient. The fact that this rhetoric comes from someone who has witnessed this inequality first-hand makes his story all the more compelling. Farmer's life story, like so many of those described in this book, is what provides the human experience and foundation for his argument. He has traveled to the poorest communities on the planet and lived side by side with those he serves. Whereas humanism advocates for focusing on the individual, Farmer might argue that you must not forsake the public health of a community for the individual patient. As physicians, we are responsible to both the individual and society, and although this relationship sometimes manifests in dilemma, it should never be far from the healer's mind. He would certainly proclaim that the rich and powerful—or perhaps the clinician who exists in a relatively powerful role in relation to the relatively vulnerable patient—must not forsake the poor and weak. His call for involvement in the bigger, global manner of advocating for equitable health care for those who cannot effectively speak for themselves cannot be rebutted by a true healer. In fact, it must be a principle by which the true healer lives his or her life.

In *Pathologies of Power*, Farmer describes in detail the many ways that the powerful take advantage of the poor. Examples of such abuses include "the cruel and unusual punishment" which is inflicted upon prisoners who suffer from tuberculosis in many parts of the world. The cruelty manifests as inmates are denied proper medical care, which leads to unavoidably increased morbidity and mortality. The high rate of this occurrence is alarming. We learn that TB transpires in prisons at rates 5–10 times the national average. And with increasing rates of TB evolves the extremely treatment-resistant strains. Drug-resistant tuberculosis is viewed, therefore, as a special form of punishment for these inmates, as they must suffer through progression of a more intense and life-threatening illness than a person given proper care. Farmer and his colleagues were invited to the Soviet Union as TB specialists in an effort to help curb this disease, which at the time was the number one cause of death in Soviet prisons. The group worked to not only improve the health for the individual patients but also improve the prisons and society as a whole. Overcrowding, poor ventilation, a lack of financial resource allocation to treat multidrug-resistant strains are but a few of the reasons for this epidemic. Farmer calls for protective public policies to help those who are victimized by this inhumane treatment. Furthermore he warns, "Transnational TB epidemics will at least remind the affluent few that as long as those epidemics remain out of control, no one is really safe" [13].

Like Edmund Pellegrino, Paul Farmer conveys how "the commodification of medical care is one of the biggest human rights issues facing the 'modern' world today" [14]. When the term "patient" is substituted by "clients" we see the commercialization of health care and the shift of the physician from healer to service-provider.[3] Farmer notes that clients (not patients) indeed are customers, someone who pays for their services. When they are viewed as such, the service in question is being defined as a commodity and not a right. Farmer is obviously repulsed by such a notion and provides many specific examples as to how this occurs, such as the fact that cancer care is almost unknown among the world's bottom billion. Farmer tells the story of one woman who was rescued from breast cancer by his organization, Partners in Health, as society turned its shoulder and otherwise left her to die from her disease. An impoverished Haitian woman was fortunate to undergo a mastectomy by a volunteering Cuban surgeon. Bridging resources across the globe, she was able to subsequently have her cancerous growth analyzed by pathologists at Brigham Women's Hospital and received chemotherapy donated by benefactors. This woman survived because of the efforts of Farmer and his colleagues as they reached above and beyond to bring her in contact with the necessary care.

To highlight the exceptional care provided by Partners in Health in Haiti, a photographic exhibit called "Structural Violence: A View From Below" was shown in Boston a few years back. One of the exhibit's guests expressed her displeasure with a photo taken by Dr. David Walton of this same poor woman, who was shown bare-chested to reveal an extensive left mastectomy scar. The entry in the guest book read, "Not appropriate at all." Farmer tells of the strife that many impoverished people undergo in the struggle to access needed health care, which is often only overcome by those with financial resources. He notes that the comment in the guest book speaks to an instinct that many in our society possess, which is to avert our gaze from things that make us uncomfortable. The guest's comment conveys an honest but unfortunate misunderstanding of intention and focuses on a superficial display of "inappropriateness" rather than seeing the beauty in this woman's survival—the fact that so many resources came together through the work of these physicians and overcame societal shortcomings to save her and others like her. Farmer concludes:

> Those who must face structural violence every day encounter precious little in the way of support for the right to food, water, housing or medical

---

[3]Carl Rogers might have a different take on this concept, which will be explored in Chap. 8.

> care ... We need to rehabilitate a series of sentiments long out of fashion in academic circles: compassion; indignation on behalf not of oneself but of the less fortunate; empathy; and even pity [14].

I initially hesitated in extending beyond discussions of the traditional clinician–patient relationship to recognize a respected belief of the healer's duty to society; however, I feel it is extremely important to acknowledge Farmer's call for the promotion of public health improvement. Dr. Martin Luther King Jr. would likely have agreed, as he once proclaimed: "Of all the forms of inequality, injustice in health care is the most shocking and inhumane." Further, it is clear that great physicians and nurses through the ages are of the same opinion. We cannot relegate our duty to our patients at large. Particularly in this age of globalization, we are more easily connected to those who are in need of health care throughout the world, and thus our ideal goals of improving social and global health are indeed reachable in a way that they were not for many centuries. I pursue a call for greater advocacy for those who are victims of inequality of health care, but do not feel intimidated by this. I do not think that anyone of us should feel guilty for practicing "conventional medicine" and serving our patients faithfully in areas where access to health care is better than other parts of the country or world. I do, however, think we are challenged to face the harsh reality that there are many others who are not getting the care they deserve and that perhaps we can do more to alleviate this disparity. Despite much advancement in medical and communication technology, this is still no easy task. I do not suggest that in order to be a consummate healer you should be willing to relocate to another country, as Schweitzer and Farmer have done. I am encouraged with the wisdom of Schweitzer who, as noted previously, recited that anyone can "have a Lambaréné." The truth is you are needed right where you are called to be. To follow are brief accounts of healers who have answered that call to serve where they are.

Unsung Heroes and Heroines

Thus far you've read about incredible feats, extraordinary deeds, and exemplary lives lived by famous healers. We can learn from their behaviors. How some of these healers lived their lives should serve as a beacon of light to those of us who may strive to "reach the unreachable star." However throughout history most of humankind has been cared for by ordinary, local clinicians who are not in the spot light. These clinicians are today's work horses who, like Maimonides, suffer silently from sheer fatigue and exhaustion seeing patients into all hours of the night. Their acts of kindness, exceptional bedside manner, astute clinical skills, and compassion are typically given without public recognition, an award, or a single honor. These are the clinicians that most fascinate me because they are uncelebrated and represent what it means to be a healer. They do the right thing when no one is watching. They behave this way because they follow their own inner compass and chart their own course without celebration. Let us now praise ordinary men and women.

Each of the healers described in this book has high character. It's important to mention that while I spend a great amount of time pointing out incredible examples of healers practicing their art, this is not to be confused with idol worship. In my research, I came across examples of human flaws found in many of those whom I have chosen to write about. Like us, they were not perfect people. I did not identify these human frailties because they are not worthy of emulating, nor are they elements of character that we should strive for. While many of the healers described herein had weaknesses, this does not mean that we cannot learn from their successes.

The Primacy of the Trusted Healing Relationship

In a previous chapter discussing the contributions of Sir William Osler, Charles S. Bryan reminds us that a clinician needs to be both competent and compassionate. However both of these admirable elements matter little if your patient doesn't trust you. According to Dr. Richard Roberts, a Professor and past Chair in the Department of Family Medicine at the University of Wisconsin Medical School in Madison, few things are as important as the "primacy of a trusted healing relationship" (Personal communication). Roberts is a highly sought-after teacher and likes to paraphrase Osler when he lectures on this topic: "more important than knowing the disease is knowing the person with the disease." Roberts further explains: "I say this because our medical 'knowledge' is often limited or suspect[4] or at

---

[4]Ioannidis JPA. Why most published research findings are false. PLoS Med. 2005;2:e124.

least fairly easy to look up. What is more important, and more difficult, is knowing the person (values, beliefs, preferences, coping style, etc.) and making a judgment about what is best for that unique person. The example I like to use is that I may be the world's greatest cardiologist and prescribe exactly the right drug for your heart, but if the odds are less than 50 % that you will ever take it correctly, or at all, (which is about what adherence rates are today), then what good have I done you?"

You and I can speculate how a patient comes to trust a physician. I am sure for some patients it is an assessment that may take as little as a few minutes. Being truthful must be a critical component. Furthermore I believe patients extend to their clinicians a line of credit. When we've pleased them we earn a credit. When we've disappointed them there is a debit from this running balance. For example, if we've worked a patient into our busy schedule who is in pain or not feeling well—that goes into our plus column. If we've made them wait (again) without as much as an apology, or made a delayed or, worse yet, incorrect diagnosis, that goes into our negative column. I think over time patients keep an unconscious running balance or assessment of our worth to them. This in turn figures into the degree of trust we are afforded.

I have personally benefitted from this trusting relationship. One of my partners in private practice had an elderly female patient whom I had developed a good rapport with over the years by virtue of our groups' custom of cross-covering for each other on weekends and holidays. I saw her 1 day for a lesion on her ear. I recommended that it be removed and she asked me if I could do it for her now. I agreed, and she was brought back to our procedure room. I used an ethyl chloride anesthetic spray to numb the upper right ear. After excising the lesion I had difficulty controlling the bleeding. Despite local pressure she continued to have a slow ooze. I decided to use the electrical cautery found on the wall behind the examining table. With one zap of the hyfrecator to her bleeding ear, her head of white hair immediately burst into flames! I put the fire out quickly by wrapping her head in the blue surgical towel on the table next to me. Apparently passing an electrical current over a volatile gas such as ethyl chloride is not a good idea. Who knew? I realized I had made a big mistake and apologized to her. After a short while she began to smile and eventually was laughing as she was getting ready to leave. On her way out the door she turned to me and said, "You know, Dr. Colgan, my son is a judge. Don't worry. I am not going to sue you." I am convinced the reason she did not pursue a complaint against me was because over time I acquired enough positive credits with her that she valued me. I've not used an electrical cautery following ethyl chloride since.

The rest of this chapter is dedicated to exemplary behaviors from unsung heroes and heroines I deeply admire. They each have earned the trust of their patients.

The Gift of Time

My personal physician gives me the impression that he has all the time in the world for me. Not only does he give me that impression— he does give me as much time as I need! My doctor listens to me. I am also fortunate that he is exceptionally bright (99 % on his board exam), evidence-based, and kind. He has both the competence and compassion Bryan writes about and was reviewed in Chap. 4.

An infectious disease doctor in my town is known as "the doctor's doctor." He is the go-to person when our hospital's physicians find themselves with an infectious disease problem. For decades he has spent very long hours walking the wards serving doctors and patients alike. Often he is called in to evaluate a patient who may be suffering from an infectious disease, but who also needs someone to just sit down and take the time to do a thorough evaluation. He lives Osler's admonition that we be thorough in our work. I often remind medical students and residents of the importance of being thorough at our morning report, when I hear they have admitted a patient to the hospital for abdominal pain and failed to do a rectal exam. Osler once remarked that "the chief function of the consultant is to make a rectal examination that you have omitted." My friend the infectious disease consultant knows this to be true. He is a true healer because of his extreme competence, compassion and because he recognizes the value of the gift of time he gives to each patient.

Muriel Petioni, a prominent Harlem physician, died this year at the age of 97. In her obituary, New York Times journalist Paul Vitello noted that she was one of the first black physicians to be given admitting privileges to Harlem hospital, breaking a tradition that forced black physicians to hand over their hospitalized patients to white physicians. She took care of the famous while never abandoning the health needs of the poor. Outside of Harlem, few probably knew

Dr. Muriel Petioni. I mention Dr. Petioni here because of a quote attributed to her by Vitello from an interview in 2011 printed in the Amsterdam News. In the quote, Dr. Petioni describes her assessment of her career: "I would give people as much time as they needed. If you had your heart and mind bursting and needed to talk to someone who was a physician, not bleeding in the body but bleeding in mind and soul, I would listen. I wasn't brilliant. I wasn't the best physician in the world, but I was nice enough to make people feel good."

Several faculty members in my department live this motto as well. They rarely ever give the sense that they are watching the clock (Although they often do run late!). The waiting room of our chairman is legendary for being full of people willing to wait hours to see him. Some have arrived without appointments. They each know that when he is with them, he is with them. He gives his patients whatever they need, and they know they are not being rushed. What a talent!

Elasticity

This is a fascinating trait that I've come to cherish in many with whom I've worked. It's the ability to be flexible and mold yourself into being that which is needed for each patient. In one room you may discern that the patient needs someone to listen, a shoulder to cry on, or a sounding board. In the next room, you may shift gears from counselor to being a skillful surgeon removing an ingrown toenail that's become terribly painful. Realizing that you must accomplish a successful nerve block so as to limit the pain associated with the procedure, you first use a small gauge needle and show patience in allowing it to work. With good surgical technique you are able to remove the nail with the least amount of discomfort. In the next room, you may come across an elderly male with multiple coronary artery disease risk factors who presents with epigastric distress. With a clenched fist to his chest he tells you "it's not a pain, really," as he waves you off. Now you are serving as a medical detective as you consider this may be an atypical presentation of acute coronary syndrome. And your day goes on. My point here is that in each scenario you are digging deep into your own clinical experience. Your clinical acumen, complemented by keeping up with the literature, enables you to give each patient what is needed when it is needed. Another example of an elastic healer is one who realizes that he/she is an introvert, but the situation at hand calls for someone personable or extroverted. Similarly, if you are by nature a bubbly, upbeat, chatty kind of person, you would show elasticity by "tuning it down" if the person across from you was depressed and admitting to thoughts of suicide.

Access

Some clinicians allow themselves to be insulated by their business phone number, fax machine, front desk, medical assistant, or other means so that there are many layers before a patient can get to them. The need to use these facilitators is entirely reasonable. I have them in place in my office. It is easy to understand how this allows you to be more efficient. I've also seen many examples of clinicians who create wide-open portals so that patients can easily get to them. This may range from providing their home or cell phone number to encouraging e-mail correspondence. Being sure that your practice has some variation of an advanced access policy is another method. Advanced access is a system whereby patients can be seen promptly once they contact your office. It's also known as open access and described as "doing today's work today." Being sure that your practice schedule is built with urgencies or acute care needs in mind is both good care and compassionate care. A healing relationship requires that you and your patient in fact see each other when necessary.

Care for the Patient

The following is an excerpt from a communication I received from a retired internist. His story is unique, yet the care he has rendered to many over the years is not. Healers like him have existed for centuries, working behind the spotlight of acclaim and recognition.

> "...a few years later one of our hospitals needed a kidney transplant program, and the nine nephrologists in town said 'no.' I suspect because they wanted to 'own it.' I went to Houston and I enlisted the help of Methodist Hospital to assist us in setting up a kidney transplant program. They said they would be happy to, they would staff it, and when we were 'up to speed' they would simply leave. The administrator and CEO of the hospital

took this information to the nephrologists… and they had a sudden change of heart. 'YES, it in fact is time to set up a transplant program.

I am no smarter than any of the subspecialists, nor the average physician. Caring, is the operative issue. My message to the young physician is 'be a real doctor, fix things that are broken, make things better, be a healer … and to be a good doctor you have to listen, be intuitive, inventive, and innovative … and pray to God for inspiration … and it will come.'"

My last story also exemplifies the trait which all healers have: they care for the patient. The woman in question is a home health nurse who looks after two home-bound patients as if they were family. She literally gets in the shower and bathes them and does whatever a loving spouse (whom they don't have) would do. She takes it upon herself to bring them to their doctors and questions these providers as if she were their daughter. She has taken them out to social venues on her own time because she knows how much it means to them. Once when she was off duty (secondary to illness) and a problem was noted in the home of her patients, she went there—pajamas underneath her regular clothing—and did what was needed. She obviously knows that "the secret in the care of the patient is to care for the patient." Not only does she care for them, she cared for them. When this section was read to her she replied, "I do love them…and they love me."

References

1. Woodward T. Make room for sentiment. Baltimore, MD: University of Maryland Medical Alumni Association; 1998.
2. Sachs J. Plato: theaetetus (focus philosophical library). Newburyport, MA: R Pullins Co.; 2004.
3. Adams F. "The oath." The genuine works of Hippocrates. Baltimore, MD: Williams and Wilkins; 1939. Trans. Francis Adams.
4. Pellegrino ED. The commodification of medical and health care: the moral consequences of a paradigm shift from a professional to a market shift. In: Engelhardt Jr H et al., editors. The philosophy of medicine reborn a Pellegrino reader. Notre Dame, IN: University of Notre Dame Press; 2008. p. 101.
5. Plato. Republic. 341c.
6. Plato. Republic. 342c.
7. Pellegrino ED. The virtues in medical practice. Oxford: Oxford University Press; 1983.
8. Pellegrino ED. Character, virtue and self interest in the ethics of the profession. In: Engelhardt Jr H et al., editors. The philosophy of medicine reborn a Pellegrino reader. Notre Dame, IN: University of Notre Dame Press; 2008. p. 135.

9. Pellegrino ED, Thomasma DC. A philosophical basis of medical practice, a philosophical reconstruction of medical morality. Oxford: Oxford University Press; 1981.
10. Largus S. Scribonii Largi Conpositiones. Edidit Georgius Helmreich. Lipsiae: BG Teubner, 1887: 2–3
11. Principles of medical ethics. American Medical Association. Jun 2001. http://www.ama-assn.org/ama/pub/physician-resources/medical-ethics/ama-code-medical-ethics/principles-medical-ethics.shtml. 10 Apr 2009
12. Review of lecture by Dr. Paul Farmer. Harvard Public Health Now. 17 Sep 2004. http://www.hsph.harvard.edu/now/sep17/program.html. 29 Mar 2009
13. Farmer P. Pathologies of power: health human rights, and the new war on the poor. Berkeley, CA: University of California Press; 2005. p. 195.
14. Farmer P. Suffering that is 'not appropriate at all'. Revista. 2003;3:42–7.

Further Reading and Resources

Pellegrino ED, Thomasma DC. A philosophical basis of medical practice. Oxford: Oxford University Press; 1981.

Pellegrino ED. Humanism and the physician. Knoxville, TN: The University of Tennessee Press; 1979.

Pellegrino ED. The virtues in medical practice. Oxford: Oxford University Press; 1983.

Kidder T. Mountains beyond mountains: the quest of Dr. Paul Farmer, a man who would cure the world. New York: Random House Trade Publications; 2004.

Farmer P. Pathologies of power: health human rights, and the new war on the poor. Berkeley, CA: University of California Press; 2005.

Farmer P. Infections and inequalities: the modern plagues. Berkeley, CA: The University of California Press; 1999.

Farmer P. The uses of Haiti. Monroe, ME: Common Courage Press; 1994.

Farmer P. AIDS and accusation: Haiti and the geography of Blame. California series in public anthropology. Berkeley, CA: The University of California Press; 1992.

Ioannidis JPA. Why most published research findings are false. PLoS Med. 2005;2:e124.

Resource

Information on partners in health, Boston, MA, can be found at www.pih.org

Part II
Practical Advice for the Modern-Day Healer

Chapter 6
Survival Tips for the Younger Clinician

The Art of Presentation

The skill of presentation is fundamental to practicing the art of medicine. While the information in this section is directed towards those in the field of medicine, nurse practitioners, nurses, and physician assistants may also benefit from reviewing this material because it is important to effectively convey the logic behind your actions, whether in writing or oral presentation. Nursing understandably uses a different form in following a different function. Examples of nursing specific communications are the patient assessment, care plan, and report. I repeatedly see students, residents, and even physicians present in a haphazard way. These people often have intelligent contributions to make to the discussion, but often their message is lost in confusion and disarray of ideas. In this section, I aim to underscore some of the crucial elements of a good presentation, so that others will appreciate how truly gifted you are.

You should begin by understanding what is expected of you, to know the basics about what factual information must be conveyed in this exchange. It is equally as important to know who will be the recipient of your message, as well as what specific format they prefer. A presentation to a cardiologist will not be the same as a presentation to an obstetrician by nature of their professional differences. Be sure you know the parlance of each specialty and what is typically looked for by different specialists. For instance, when presenting patient information to a cardiologist, you must be sure to know all the coronary artery disease (CAD) risk factors of your patient, as well as

R. Colgan, *Advice to the Healer: On the Art of Caring*,
DOI 10.1007/978-1-4614-5170-9_6,
© Springer Science+Business Media, LLC 2013

previous cardiac catheterization details. If your patient has chest pain, be sure to include the descriptors of angina too. Be mindful how often patients with coronary artery disease present without classical angina. I have been impressed how often I've heard patients tell me "it's not a pain really" while waving their hand from left to right in an attempt to dismiss my concern. An obstetrician is going to want to know your patient's last menstrual period, menstrual cycle characteristics, and gestational history. Regardless of the specialty, there are some critical facts that must always be accounted for and reported. Look to understand upfront if you are being asked to give a full comprehensive presentation, e.g., a formal morning report or if a 1-minute, "tell me who you admitted last night," description is expected.

Young healers typically get a brief rundown on how to properly present a patient and are encouraged to describe this information in a certain order. Often this education is inadequate, and they learn shortly after how they screwed something up—how they should have put this in the history of present illness (HPI) or left something else out of the analysis, etc. It is important to learn how to present a patient efficiently and thoroughly for three reasons. First, if you follow Osler's admonition of developing a particular method, you will consciously do things the same way each time and are less likely to forget something of significance. If you always order your presentation as chief complaint, history of present illness, past medical history, current medications, then allergies, you are less likely to ever forget to ask your patient if they are allergic to something and even less likely to prescribe a medicine that may result in a fatal allergic reaction. Implicit for a good presentation is that you have performed your evaluation in a thorough manner and that you have followed a proper method. For example, present the history with proper method by recounting the patient's story in a chronological and descriptive manner. Start at the beginning "when did your problem begin, in other words: when were you last well." Present the physical exam with proper method by logically displaying information from head to toe.

Second, it is important to present effectively so that your listener, typically a fellow clinician, can clearly understand what you did or plan to do. A good presentation will enable a subsequent care provider to easily pick up where you left off and provide a smooth transition to enable the best possible patient care. A good presentation is not a comprehensive data dump, where you look to impress the listener with the fact that you asked everything. A good presentation is giving the listener the significant information they need to know so as to be able to understand what you learned, have input into the case, and perhaps eventually take over that person's care. An example of an improper patient presentation is calling your attending at two in the morning to give an overly thorough description of your stable patient's entire health history including his banana allergy. (This actually happened to me!) You should succinctly give your listeners the information they need to make their own independent assessment as to what is going on with the patient. This part is slightly tricky, because it implies that you know all of the pertinent positive and negative questions and answers to include in your presentation—which as a young healer you may not. You are learning these as you pursue your training and will continue to learn more and more each day of your career. Like any other skill, the discovery and recognition of significant information comes with practice.

Third, you should strive to learn how to present well, because it is the language of medicine. The listener is often going to evaluate and assume your competence based in part on how well you use the language of medicine—in short, how well you presented. To be blunt, you can be brilliant yet present badly, and your mentor will think you to be disorganized or incompetent. The sooner you master the skill of presentation, the sooner you will impress all of those who listen to you and earn recognition as someone who is organized and coherent. You will more likely be viewed as competent. Let me go over a few rules:

In giving a presentation you simply start at the beginning, which is always the chief complaint. This is best given in the patient's own words and not your assessment of what he or she meant. In other words, say that the patient stated, "I couldn't breathe" rather than, "The patient presented with shortness of breath or dyspnea." The chief complaint is always followed by the history of present illness (HPI). This is the most important part of the entire history, so you want to be very careful that you attend to it well. Begin by describing the patient, e.g., "This is the first university hospital admission for this 24-year-old African American female who was last well until the evening prior to admission when she noted she couldn't breathe." The HPI should read like a newspaper article, wherein the most important sentence—or the lead—is first and then subsequently followed by more detailed information of lesser importance. Like a good journalist, do not bury your lead! Do not hide a critical piece of historical information further down in the body of the report, when in fact it is crucial to understanding the patient's illness. For instance, if your patient was also suffering from an underlying malignancy, was on oral contraceptive therapy, and her shortness of breath occurred simultaneously with the abrupt onset of a dry cough on the day after her long airplane flight, which was 1 week after she had her left leg placed in a cast for a chip fracture of the ankle that occurred while skiing, say so. She may have pulmonary emboli, and as you present your patient in a logical and prioritized fashion, you will help your colleague better understand how you achieved that conclusion. Although each piece of information could theoretically be categorized under many different parts of the patient's history, they are details that are extremely important in deciphering the case. It is up to you to recognize them as such and give them to your listener as coherently and concisely as possible.

In your HPI, present your data methodically and chronologically in a continuum from when the patient felt well to the present sick condition. Follow your HPI with past medical history, medications, and allergies. For example, "The patient is allergic to codeine and suffered anaphylactic shock when she took it in the past." Even if a nurse or medical assistant has filled this information in for you, you should personally ask each patient about medications and allergies. Do this every time you see a patient, for the rest of your life. To not do so is bad practice, and mistakes made by missing this opportunity to collect and/or confirm valuable patient information can harm your patient and your career. This is a good template for the most essential components of the subjective portion of your presentation. Remember to collect as much information as possible. If asked, you should be prepared to provide supplemental facts from the family history, social history, and review of systems, while realizing that pertinent information should already have been mentioned in the HPI.

The objective exam should always begin with your patient's general appearance followed by his or her vital signs. The general appearance should be such that you could easily pick the patient from a crowd of people or a waiting room. Remember that the vital signs are… vital. In fact they are arguably, along with the general appearance, the most important signs under the objective portion of your presentation. Yet these two descriptors are often given little to no mention. You can be brief in saying that your patient "looks to be in no acute distress and is with stable vital signs." Just be sure to include some recognition of this valuable information. Also, as with the history of present illness, make sure to mention significant vital signs when they apply directly. If our theoretical patient was suffering from pulmonary emboli, we would want to specifically mention her respiratory rate and if she appeared to be in any respiratory distress, followed by her pulse oximetry reading. Almost every patient you care for in the clinical practice of medicine, certainly in primary care medicine, should have his or her heart and lungs auscultated. Granted, there may be some particular exceptions to this rule; but most physicians should listen to their patient's heart and lungs at each visit. This is not necessarily for the purpose of discovering some pathology — not to search for a mid-systolic click or pick up subtle bronchophony — but so you may lay your hands on the patient. Every great healer knows the value of (appropriately) touching your patient. You should go out of your way to practice a "laying on of the hands." It is part of a therapeutic, professional intimacy between physician and patient, a conveyance of compassion for the person you are providing care. It is a sign, at a minimum, of *kindness*. Lastly, be sure to comment on "the other" or anything else in the physical exam that may be noteworthy. In our patient above, you may also comment that you do or do not hear a fixed splitting of the second heart sound as might be heard in massive pulmonary emboli.

After your objective exam comes the hardest part for physicians in training: the assessment and plan. It is the most challenging, for the less clinical training you have experienced the less ability you possess to develop a broad differential diagnosis. The assessment should not be a repetition of your history and physical. It should be your synthesis of a working diagnosis, even if you do not know what is going on. Continuing our example: If you are not sure what is causing your patient's shortness of breath, you should list what you know as fact: "Problem number one is dyspnea, etiology unclear. Problem number two is recent left leg fracture. Problem number three is previous codeine anaphylaxis, and problem number four is health maintenance — it is noted that it has been several years since her last pap smear." Call your patient's problem what you understand it to be at the time. Other examples might be "chest pain, etiology unclear" or "vesicular unilateral T5 dermatomal eruption, etiology unclear." By stating your working diagnosis, you know where you are and are given a lead as to how to proceed. Also, it communicates to your listener that the gears are turning, and you are thinking along a logical train of thought, even if you have not yet arrived at the answer.

Lastly is your plan. This plan should be congruent with your assessment. If you have mentioned three active problems in your assessment, you should have three active plan items. The plan also includes patient education goals, prescription of medications, and diagnostics including any additional studies you would like to order. In addition, every time you see patients it is wise to include in your plan what they can do to help themselves, as well as when they should contact you again and return for care. Some variations to this apply. If you are seeing a patient for an acute or sick visit, there should be some mention of health maintenance under his or her assessment or plan. This is your opportunity to inquire if he/she is up to date on age-appropriate health screenings, e.g., an annual well-woman exam. If not, part of your plan should be a recommendation that your patient also consider making an appointment for whatever health screening exams they require. In continuing with the example of our clinical case of a young woman with shortness of breath, our plan might have the following components: "(1) Explained to patient my concern for life threatening pulmonary emboli; she agrees to emergency department transfer by ambulance for consideration of imaging studies to rule out pulmonary emboli; (2) Continued non-weight bearing and use of crutches in light of her recent leg fracture; (3) Avoid codeine given allergy to same; consider non-steroidal anti-inflammatory for pain relief; and (4) Patient urged to make a follow-up visit at a later date for a well-woman exam." One of my partners in private practice taught me that in his residency they encouraged physicians to include under plan, in addition to what was discussed above, any recommendations about diet, exercise, and stress. Hippocrates would be proud.

Common mistakes occur as presentations become disorganized and messy. Your presentation should start with the subjective ("S" What did your patient say?), followed by the objective ("O" What did you observe, auscultate, palpate, percuss… find?), followed by your assessment ("A" What do you think is going on?) and finally your plan ("P" What are you going to do?). A common mistake that all physicians in training and young physicians make is going from topic to topic, or from "S" to "P" to "A" to "O" to "S" to "O" to "S" again, back to "P," etc. My advice to you is to tell them the "S," the pertinent

"S," and nothing but the "S." Then pause. Indent your presentation so the listener knows you are now leaving "the land of S," for the "land of O." When you get to "O," always begin with general appearance, followed by those most vital signs. (They are vital!) When young healers get to the assessment they often want to repeat the "S" and "O" again. You must fight hard not to do this and continue on to "A" and "P" by laying out the patient's problems and attempted solutions. My advice to the young healer is to practice your presentation skills as often as you can and be thankful when a senior clinician "pokes you in the ribs" and tells you to do it differently. You must always strive to be the best communicator of medicine possible. In the end, the patient will be better served, you will be a better physician, and you will be viewed in a more mature light.

Practice Makes for Better Practice

A common lament of the younger clinician is the misunderstanding that you have to know it all. Even the best-seasoned clinicians start out young, green, naïve, with little clinical experience. When I chose to go into private practice, I specifically sought out a group of several doctors older than myself thinking that I would be able to learn from them. I was not disappointed. But even then I did not know how much I didn't know. I was surprised when the venerable and wise senior physician of our group told me shortly after my arrival, "Don't worry—in about 10 years you'll get in your groove." I was astounded to think that it would take 10 years. But he was right, i.e., the longer you practice medicine, the better you get at it. Another academic physician who had been practicing for 25 years told me of being urged by his wife to give up obstetrics. When asked why he decided to stay in the field he reasoned, "I am just getting good at it."

The young healer must understand that you are not required to know it all during your studies, upon graduation from professional school, or even through further training. But once you are practicing on your own, you are responsible for knowing what you know and being humble enough to acknowledge what you do not know in order to practice the standard of care. One of the best skills to develop as a young healer is the capacity to say, "I don't know." After which, of course, must follow the conscious reflection of evaluating the situation and deciding how next to proceed. This may seem difficult on the surface, but really simplifies to the question of whether or not the given situation, in the clinical area you are unfamiliar with, is or is not an emergency. If you come upon a victim of a motor vehicle accident on the side of the road and blood is shooting from his carotid artery: apply compression. This is an emergency! If it is an emergency—or the patient's airway, breathing, or circulation is compromised—call for immediate help. Short of situations as dire as this, most everything else is either urgent or elective. Urgent matters can be clarified by talking with a colleague, picking up the phone, referring to a textbook, or looking something up on the Internet. An urgent clinical issue implies that if you do not attend to the matter promptly harm may be done to the patient. In the earlier clinical case scenario, the young female patient who presented to the ski patrol with a painful swollen ankle (and not yet with chest pain or shortness of breath) could be categorized as someone in need of urgent care. She should have her ankle problem addressed promptly. As opposed to urgent problems, elective problems can generally wait a while to be attended to, such as the fact that she was overdue for her well-woman exam. Elective clinical problems are those in which you are unsure of how to next proceed, and these can typically wait until you obtain the information you need to make an appropriate decision. A decision to start a cholesterol-lowering agent in a patient for whom you are unclear as to the proper application of the latest recommendations for drug interactions can wait until you have the chance to check the literature.

In researching for this book, I spoke to many physicians and contacted colleagues who I personally hold in high esteem to gain their insights on the art of caring. I asked them who they considered exemplary figures throughout history, those who practiced the art of caring in a manner to which we all should aspire. Many shook their heads and let their voices trail off after naming only one or two figures. But when I asked doctors how it was they learned the art of medicine, most replied that the greatest lessons came from working alongside a revered mentor. Although lessons on the art of medicine as taught by "ordinary healers" is not the theme of this book, the truth is that all of us look to role models for the types of behavior we want to emulate. This modeling of good practices is one of the most important ways we learn the art of medicine. We practice it and inspire those around us to do the same. "The Practice of Medicine is an art based on a science," Osler tells us [1]. It entails skills and crafts that we learn from seeing others do it. "See one, do one, teach one" is an adage that most interns have heard. This applies not only to procedure—directing how to put in an intravenous line or drain an abscess—but also to many of the softer, subtler ways that physicians practice their craft, their *art*.

When I was a third-year resident, I remember doing a rotation with Dr. J. Roy Guyther in Mechanicsville, Maryland. Dr. Guyther is one of Maryland's giants in family medicine, who helped develop the specialty from the horse and buggy general practitioner to the current residency-trained family physician. I did not expect to learn so much about evidence-based medicine and the art of its practice from my grey-haired mentor, and I am fortunate to have shared many experiences with him. I recall one memorable moment in particular: I was watching Dr. Guyther help an elderly woman on a particularly busy afternoon. She arrived with a litany of complaints, all of which he addressed, and this caused him to be even further behind than he already was. Thinking the extended visit was finally over, he walked toward the door. The patient said, "Dr. Guyther, there is… one more thing." "What is that," he replied, to which she answered "I'd like to talk to you about my constipation." I never expected what happened next. Dr. Guyther returned to his seat, and over the next several minutes he actually took the time to listen to her concerns, ask more details, and help her with her problem. These "oh by the way" questions, also known as the "hand on the doorknob" concerns, occur quite often and can be a significant source of stress for the physician as they are interpreted as an inconvenience or obligation. Often, if physicians do not take the time to address these concerns, the patient interaction is rushed and incomplete. But in this situation, Dr. Guyther modeled considerate patient care for me, and this has been just as significant in my medical education as those who have shown me the proper procedure to obtain an arterial blood gas. Although the time for this assistance was not in his schedule, Dr. Guyther made the time because the patient needed him. He selflessly attended to his patient and provided her with exceptional care.

These instances of phenomenal patient care can be as simple as the one above or may be life-altering. Dr. Edward Kowalewski, one of the founding fathers of the American Academy of Family Physicians and the first Chair of the Department of Family and Community Medicine at the University of Maryland, proved that taking the necessary time to provide thorough and expert care can truly change the patient's life. A patient once sought Dr. Kowalewski's help in an office visit, during which he disclosed that he had just killed another man. As the story goes, Dr. Kowalewski installed a switch that could be activated from his exam room desk, which turned on a "do not disturb" red light outside the room. Ninety minutes after having indicated that he did not want to be interrupted during this patient visit, the two men emerged from the consultation and walked to the police station, where the patient turned himself into authorities. Observing "ordinary" healers doing extraordinary things for their patients is how many seasoned clinicians describe their experience of learning the essentials of the physician–patient relationship. We learn to be better healers not only through diligent study and committed practice but by seeking out mentors and striving to model exceptional behaviors. Their lessons have withstood the test of time and should not be forgotten.

Good Communication

Communication is an essential skill required for any person with ambitions to become a great healer. One of the leading reasons why patients complain about their doctors is a lack of explanation and poor communication [2]. Poor communication between the physician and patient has been shown to be a factor in malpractice litigation [3]. So while hopefully we can agree that good communication is necessary and valuable, this begs the question: How can we learn how to better communicate with our patients? We all think we know good communication when we hear it, but how do you practice it?

In May 1999, 21 leaders and representatives from major medical education and professional organizations attended an invitational conference in Kalamazoo, Michigan with the goal of delineating a coherent set of essential elements in physician–patient communication [4]. The participants wanted to devise a short list of elements to characterize effective communication, provide tangible examples of skill competencies that would be useful to medical educators at all levels, and be both evidence-based and amenable to assessment and evaluation.

The end product of the Bayer-Fetzer Conference on Patient–Physician Communication in Medical Education is summarized below.

The Kalamazoo Consensus Statement [4]

Essential Elements of Communication in Medical Encounters

1. *Build a relationship.* Develop a patient-centered or relationship-centered approach to care. Strive to build a partnership with your patient, while realizing that the patient's ideas and values maybe different than your own.
2. *Open the discussion.* Hear what the patient has to say in his or her own words, attempting to understand what he or she may be worried about, while making a connection with your patient.
3. *Gather information.* Use open-ended and closed-ended questions to better understand what is going on; try to clarify what you need to know and summarize what you think you understand, while actively listening to the patient using nonverbal and verbal techniques.
4. *Understand the patient's perspective.* Try to understand your patient's background better, e.g., family, cultural, socioeconomic, and spiritual, inquiring as to his or her beliefs and concerns and what the patient hopes to achieve from his or her visit with you.
5. *Share information.* Be sure that you are communicating with your patient in a manner that can be easily understood, e.g., avoiding medical terminology that may be misunderstood and being mindful of his or her educational background. Afterwards, the committee advises checking back with your patients to see if they understood what you were trying to convey and if they had any additional questions.
6. *Reach agreement.* Develop a consensus between you and your patient as to how you will both proceed, while enlisting resources and supports that may help you both.
7. *Provide closure.* And lastly, determine if your patient has any additional concerns, summarizing what you understand to be your conjoint plan and discussing when you should meet again.

Gregory Makoul, Ph.D., Chief Academic Officer and Senior Vice President for Innovation and Quality Integration at St. Francis Hospital in Hartford, Connecticut provided leadership in writing the Kalamazoo statement and has also offered another article containing a mnemonic that some may find helpful in remembering some of the above techniques [5]. The SEGUE framework for teaching and assessing communication skills stands for: Set the stage, Elicit information, Give information, Understand the patient's perspective, and End the encounter.

Good communication and clinical judgment are critical talents for the aspiring healer to achieve. You may have a brilliant intellect, effectively practice evidence-based medicine, and show great consideration for your patient. But if you cannot clearly and efficiently convey your clinical impression to a colleague or your patient, you will be undervalued and the physician–patient relationship will not nearly be as rich or satisfactory. Presenting a patient properly, effectively communicating with your patient, and maintaining sound clinical judgment are talents which we are not born with but must learn and develop over time. If you feel like you are not where you want to be in this regard, that is a good sign. It means you recognize that you can do better—and you will. Throughout your transition from technician to healer, keep in mind that every mentor you have ever looked up to, every person you view as being exemplary in the practice of medicine began his or her clinical career as a young physician just like you.

References

1. The Osler Society of New York. http://www.oslersociety.org/index.php/by-osler
2. Vincent C, et al. Why do people sue doctors? Lancet. 1994;343:1609–13.
3. Beckman H, Markakis K, Suchman AL, Frankel R. The doctor-patient relationship and malpractice: lessons from plaintiff depositions. Arch Intern Med. 2000;154:1365–70.
4. Participants in the Bayer-Fetzer Conference on Physician-Patient Communication in Medical Education. Essential elements of communication in medical encounters: the Kalamazoo consensus statement. Acad Med. 2001;76(4):390–3.
5. Makoul G. The SEGUE framework for teaching and assessing communication skills. Patient Educ Couns. 2001;45(1):23–4.

How to Present

A guide to improving presentation of oral cases can be found at the site below: <http://depts.washington.edu/medclerkhj/student/presentation.html>
In addition, Loyola University provides an instructional video about "Oral Presentation on Rounds," accessible below: <www.medicalvideos.us/play.php?vid=740>

Practice Makes for Better Practice

Selzer R. Letters to a young doctor. Boston, MA: Mariner Books; 1996.
Groopman J. How doctors think. Boston, MA: Mariner Books; 2008.

Chapter 7
Civility

A healer must uphold a professional, considerate, and kind manner during all interactions with his or her patients. This notion applies from the time of introduction and initial exam, through follow-up consults, visits with family members, and any other patient encounter. Hippocrates explains how physicians should compose themselves from the very moment they meet the patient. In *Decorum*, we are taught upon entering a patient's room to "bear in mind [our] manner of sitting, reserve, arrangement of dress, decisive utterance, brevity of speech, composure, bedside manners, (and) care" [1]. Dr. Michael W. Kahn, a psychiatrist from Beth Israel Deaconess Medical Center and assistant professor of psychiatry at Harvard Medical School, published an article in the *New England Journal of Medicine* which highlights our patients' desires and expectations to be treated by doctors that are well behaved [2]. I think the lessons of this study are applicable to all clinicians. As thoughtful practitioners, we are well aware of the humanistic and caring qualities that are required for the most effective health care delivery. However, Kahn speculates that many "patients may care less about whether their doctors are reflective and empathic than whether they are respectful and attentive" [2]. Dr. Kahn notes that most patients complain not of being misunderstood or denied empathy but rather of physician behaviors they perceive as rude or neglectful. Dr. Kahn believes that good manners can be learned; moreover, he elucidates how physicians should be reminded to cultivate these behaviors so as to practice "etiquette-based medicine" [2].

R. Colgan, *Advice to the Healer: On the Art of Caring*,
DOI 10.1007/978-1-4614-5170-9_7,
© Springer Science+Business Media, LLC 2013

Dr. Kahn explains how it is simpler to change physician behavior than patient attitudes:

> Etiquette-based medicine would prioritize behavior over feeling. It would stress practice and mastery over character development. It would put professionalism and patient satisfaction at the center of the clinical encounter and bring back some of the elements of ritual that have always been an important part of the healing professions [2].

There have evolved many behaviors that are not only expected by the patient, but are seen as standards of care by many institutions. Thus, there has evolved many suggestions for physicians providing care to hospitalized patients to act in a way that is valued by patients. The following checklist, also reported in the *New York Times*, offers six simple behaviors that are shown to be perceived by the patient as professional and attentive [3].

The Six Habits of Highly Respectful Physicians

1. Ask permission to enter the room and wait for an answer before doing so.
2. Introduce yourself, showing your ID badge.
3. Shake hands with your patient (wear gloves if needed).
4. Sit down and smile if appropriate.
5. Briefly explain your role on the patient's health care team.
6. Ask the patient how he or she is feeling about being in the hospital and listen to the response.

Etiquette-based medicine is such a simple, obvious necessity in the practice of medicine. So much so, that you almost have to wonder why it is being promoted at all. Isn't this already the standard of care? Don't physicians aspire to practice medicine through good behavior? The answers to these questions are not straightforward and are unfortunately compounded by the sad reality that these simple expectations are not always met. Etiquette-based medicine is *not* uniformly practiced today. This lack of civility is not unique to medicine, but an insidious social problem that has escalated over time according to Dr. P.M. Forni, a professor at Johns Hopkins University and cofounder of the Johns Hopkins Civility Project. In Dr. Forni's book *Choosing Civility* he makes the suggestion that "we agree on one principle: that a crucial measure of our success in life is the way we treat one another every day of our lives" [4]. Dr. Forni cites 25 behaviors which the civil person exemplifies. Most of these "rules" are important considerations for all members of society and are applicable to clinicians as we strive to become the most effective civil healers possible. Those who wish to improve their healing skills may adapt some of these rules in the care of the patient. The 25 "rules" are included below with examples of how they may relate to patient care.

The 25 Rules of Considerate Conduct Abridged for the Healer

1. *Pay attention.* This is understood as a variation of Hippocrates urging that we observe all and of Osler's admonition to use all of our senses when caring for the patient.
2. *Acknowledge others.* Introducing ourselves to others in the room and understanding how they may be familiar with our patient is an example of acknowledging others.
3. *Think the best.* It is easy to assume that a patient requesting narcotics is drug seeking, when in fact the patient likely wants relief from a physical or emotional pain. Our challenge is to begin each encounter with a hopeful attitude and optimistic expectations. We must be careful not to pre-judge patients, even though it is known that some patients may be drug seeking.
4. *Listen.* We have already learned that if you listen to the patients, they will tell you the diagnosis, and that much can be inferred from non-verbal communications. I observed a great example of a clinician who showed a keen sense of listening. Recently, in explaining an unpleasant event to a colleague and several third-year medical students, the attending took a long deep breath, followed by a long audible exhalation. In observing this, the astute medical student acknowledged a "deep sigh" gaining information on the attending's mood, opinions, and emotional state that may have not otherwise been obvious from words alone. I was impressed because she showed astute listening skills—not only to the spoken word but to other sounds around her.
5. *Be inclusive.* Certainly the best way we can be inclusive in the medical profession is by honoring cultural diversity through

considerate and thoughtful medical practice. An example of this would be asking our patients who are having sex if that is with men, women or both.

6. *Speak kindly.* Beginning your interview with something like, "How may I help?" and ending with a simple, "Is there anything else I can do for you?" denotes kindness.

7. *Do not speak ill.* Healers are at their best when they do not criticize the care rendered by others. Doing so sabotages our common mission of helping the patient.

8. *Accept and give praise.* One of the best ways to promote well-being in our patients is to go out of our way to find something positive in what they have done to positively affect their health and then compliment them for doing so. Encouraging our patients, and having what the American psychologist Carl Rogers calls "unconditional positive regard" is something we can easily do to improve our patient's health care experience (See Chap. 8).

9. *Respect even a subtle "no."* Of course we must respect our patient's wishes when they do not agree with our recommendations; however, we still have an obligation to obtain proper informed consent with respect to what may happen if a patient does not follow our advice. It is our duty to provide the patient with all the information necessary to make an educated decision about his or her health. Even in dire circumstances—such as disregarding advice to visit the emergency department when experiencing anginal chest pain—the patient must understand the consequences. Although difficult, it is our obligation to lay down the facts, especially when disregarding professional medical advice may result in the patient's death; after which, if the answer is still "no," we must respect and honor that person's wishes.

10. *Respect other's opinions.* This works in all directions in every relationship in health care. A primary care provider must value the opinions of a consultant, just as a consultant must value the opinions of his or her primary care colleague. We must value the opinions of our patients, with the hope that they will value ours. Understanding these dynamic relationships and being aware of their implications for health care delivery will serve our patients well.

11. *Mind your body.* We cannot take good care of our patients if we do not take good care of ourselves. Often the physician puts his or her health to the wayside to accomplish his or her professional duties. We will explore this further in a later in chapter 10, in a section called Heal Thyself.

12. *Be agreeable.* Even though we may disagree with our patient's decision, we must strive to be agreeable and continue to help in the most effective way possible in the context of that disagreement. As with the example in number nine, although we may not agree with the decision to forego emergency room care, we can still be agreeable. We can agree to disagree in a civil manner.

13. *Keep it down (and rediscover silence).* Psychiatrists seem to have cornered the market on appreciating the value of silence. This is a skill which, when appropriate, we can emulate. Much can be gained from silence. Often, giving the anxious patient an extended period of time to think before they respond to a question will result in information that may have been missed. Be patient, do not assume, and listen. Allowing our patients their time to tell us what is concerning to them is civility at its best.

14. *Respect other people's time.* "Running late" is at the top of most patients' lists of what frustrates them during visits to their doctor's office. Often this is the reality of health care delivery, as unexpected situations arise and simply take longer than expected. However, we can try to prevent dissatisfaction through our actions such as being on time to the office, not overbooking inordinately, and—when all else fails—simply apologizing when we are late. This occurred for me recently when I assumed the role of the patient. I had an appointment with a highly respected and very busy physician and still had not been called back to the room 45 min after my appointed time. I had another meeting to attend, so I informed his front desk staff that I needed to reschedule. Although I realized he must have had an urgent situation arise, I was displeased that I had wasted 2 h of my time. I was surprised to answer a call from this physician at 5:30 that night, apologizing for keeping me waiting. This simple gesture showed class and respect.

15. *Respect other people's space.* It is proper to ask for permission to sit down or start an exam when visiting a hospitalized patient.

16. *Apologize earnestly.* We are going to make mistakes in the course of our job. When we do, it is appropriate and necessary to apologize. Gallagher and colleagues reported in a 2003 JAMA article on patients' and physicians' attitudes regarding the disclosure of medical errors that "physicians should strive to meet patients' desires for an apology and for information on the nature, cause, and prevention of errors" [5].

17. *Assert yourself.* Our duty is to assert ourselves for our patients, especially when doing so will result in more comprehensive care.

This is not always easy or glamorous and often is the source of conflict—such as appealing for a previously denied authorization for medical care by an insurance company or going to extra lengths to make sure proper information about your patient reaches a consultant. We should all strive to be the physician that "goes the extra mile" for his or her patients.

18. *Avoid (unnecessary) personal questions.* Our job description entails asking personal questions as part of a true physician–patient interaction. The medical consultation room is sometimes referred to as "the confessional," because it is behind these closed doors in which our patients will tell us things they may never tell anyone else. It is a privilege to be in a position to gather this information; furthermore, to possess such trust and patient confidence. Personal questions are needed to gather pertinent information for patient diagnosis, treatment, and follow-up care. The patient's personal history often has important medical implications. However, this does not give us license to ask personal questions beyond medical necessity to satisfy our own curiosity. While it may be important to ascertain if a patient is receiving social security disability income, medical assistance, food stamps, or the like, it would likely not be necessary to ask someone who by all appearances is not financially depressed about how much money they make. It is our professional duty to use personal information where appropriate and not overstep our privilege by asking inappropriate or irrelevant questions.

19. *Care for your guests.* It is important to have an office that is accommodating to our elderly and disabled patients; moreover, when extra assistance is provided, it should be done so with respect and thoughtfulness.

20. *Be a considerate guest.* When conducting a home visit, we should schedule our appointment at a time that is amenable to both the care provider *and* the patient. In the course of the home visit, we must be respectful of their environment. For example, asking for permission to sit in a certain chair, use a certain area for the exam, or wash your hands on the way out shows great consideration.

21. *Think twice before asking for favors.* The physician–patient relationship represents a complex distribution of power. We are a profession of power—gatekeepers to medical information and health services—and help those who are vulnerable. It can be safely argued that we should not, in the course of our caring for patients, ask for favors from them.

22. *Refrain from idle complaints.* There is no room in our practice for complaints. Common ones such as "the office has overbooked me again," or "the insurance companies keep wringing me dry," or "I am not paid enough for what I do" are known frustrations associated with providing medical care. However, it does no good to practice with such negative attitudes. We must always realize that as bad as we think things may be for us, they are typically much, much worse for those whom we serve.

23. *Accept and give constructive criticism.* Some of the most valuable lessons we can learn come from our patients as they offer criticism of our care. We should remember that neither the overly flattering nor the overly critical patient is likely accurate in assessing our overall care. But we can learn from frank comments from our patients. Likewise, we can and should learn from constructive criticism from our colleagues and teachers. However, it is important to be objective when doing so and not make personal attacks or take criticism personally. Many young physicians may feel disheartened when they receive criticism, but it is important to realize this is because your mentor believes in you and wants to help you be the best you can be. We all will make mistakes and are expected to learn from them. I have witnessed many examples of constructive or necessary criticism that often leaves the young clinicians feeling embarrassed. Some of these include the admonition to refrain from chewing gum while seeing a patient as it denotes an air of casualness to the physician–patient visit. Some may be not so obvious: do not look at your cell phone or text messages while in the exam room with your mentor. Do not sit at the ambulatory care center desk when work is slow and listen to music via headphones, feet up on a chair as if you are at home. Do not arrive more than 30 min late for your patient care session—with a valid reason, of course—without calling in advance to give notice. Another very important criticism I have reinforced to many students throughout the years is not following through when say you are going to do something, such as follow-up on a test, an outstanding report, or a phone call. As Dr. Woodward (see Chap. 5) would remind you, "Your word is your bond."

24. *Respect the environment and be gentle to animals.* Schweitzer (see Chap. 5) might use this rule to advocate for reverence for life—all life.

25. *Don't shift responsibility and blame.* When I became the medical director of the Family Medicine Department, I took over

responsibilities for an academic health center that serves close to 40,000 patients per year. I learned a terrific lesson from the practice manager, called the "Triple A approach." The Triple A approach is useful in dealing with a patient who is angry because of a perceived wrong inflicted upon him or her by you or your organization. If appropriate, you can often quickly diffuse a volatile situation by (1) Acknowledging that the person is upset, (2) Accepting responsibility (if and when it is yours to own), and (3) Amending the situation as best you can.

I have an example from my own career that illustrates this technique. I once walked into an examination room to be greeted by the glaring stare of a patient whom I admitted to our local hospital at 2 a.m. for an acute myocardial infarction, and was greeted by his glaring stare. After a few minutes of speaking to him with his arms folded on his chest and his muscles tense, I said to him, "You look angry." He nodded and said, "Yes, I am." When I asked him why he felt this way, he eventually opened up and asked if I remembered examining him in the emergency department. Feeling good about the fact that we diagnosed his acute infarction in time to give him thrombolytic therapy and heparin I said, "Yes, I remember." Then he asked me, "Why did you stick your finger in my behind?" Apparently, unbeknownst to me, my patient was angry that I performed a standard rectal exam (so as to be sure he was not with an occult gastrointestinal bleed that might preclude the safe use of anticoagulation therapy). I realized that I must have done a poor job of explaining why it was necessary to do this exam and failed to convey how it was standard practice of care that would be conducted for any other patient in his situation. He felt violated. After acknowledging his anger, I accepted responsibility for not explaining to him why this particular exam was important. I then looked to make amends by promising him that I would attempt to be more careful in the future with other patients, should this situation ever arise again. At the end of the visit we were friendly with each other again—but I learned a valuable lesson about proper communication from this encounter. More importantly, I accepted responsibility for my patient's dissatisfaction and changed my behavior in future practice to avoid its reoccurrence.

The works of Drs. Kahn and Forni are critical in understanding how best to practice the art of caring for others. While it is important to be competent, altruistic, virtuous, well-meaning, and all of the other character traits that constitute a clinician successful in practicing the art of caring, these authors highlight the need to translate good training, intentions, and medical practice into behaviors that are perceived by the patient as being proper, civil, respectful, and professional. You might consider taking an inventory of how you are going to be respectful before you visit your next patient as impractical or obvious, but, from my experience, I do not think our patients feel this way. If anything, patients are impressed by such attention to detail regarding their satisfaction of care. Osler (see Chap. 5) might have argued that you are faithfully following two of his cardinal teachings: method and thoroughness. If each of us were competent in practicing etiquette-based medicine and did so at all times, we would not need to be reminded of this. But if we are honest with ourselves, we may admit that there are times when fatigue, inattentiveness, and maybe just being rushed have led to patient interactions that are less civil than our personal ideals. Be aware of yourself, your patients, and how your behaviors, actions, and mannerisms affect their health care experiences.

References

1. Adams F. The genuine works of Hippocrates, Williams and Wilkins, Baltimore, 1939.
2. Kahn M. Etiquette based medicine. N Engl J Med. 2008;358:1988–9.
3. Kahn M. The six habits of highly respectable physicians. late ed. New York Times. Dec 3 2008.
4. Forni P. Choosing civility: the 25 rules of considerate conduct. New York: St. Martin's Griffin; 2002.
5. Gallagher T, Waterman A. Patients and physicians' attitudes regarding the disclosure of medical errors. JAMA. 2003;289:1001–7.

Civility

Small J, et al. Improving your bedside manner: a handbook for physicians to develop therapeutic conversations with their patient. Austin, TX: Eupsychian Press; 2008.

Cassell EJ. The healers art. Cambridge, MA: The MIT Press; 1985.

Moise H. Physician-patient relations: a guide to improving satisfaction. Chicago, IL: American Medical Association Press; 1999.

Ludwig J. Physician-patient relationship. University of Washington School of Medicine. 11 Apr 2008. <http://depts.washington.edu/bioethx/topics/physpt.html>. Accessed 30 Apr 2009.

Defining the patient-physician relationship for the 21st Century. American Healthways and Johns Hopkins 3rd Annual disease Management Outcomes Summit. Phoenix, AZ. 30 Oct 2003. <http://www.patient-physician.com/docs/PatientPhysician.pdf>. Accessed 30 Apr 2009.

Owens D. Hospitality to strangers: empathy and the physician-patient relationship. Atlanta, GA: American Academy of Religion Book; 1999.

Chapter 8
Lessons Learned from Private Practice

The Clinician as Counselor

Counseling using therapeutic techniques is an essential part of being
a good clinician. Carl R. Rogers was one of the most influential psychologists in American history and pioneered the concept of having
unconditional positive regard when counseling a patient. Unconditional
positive regard involves showing complete support and acceptance of
a person no matter what that person says or does. One way to incorporate unconditional positive regard is to look at every clinical
encounter and ask what you can do that would be uplifting, supportive, nurturing and show kindness to your patient. This may be challenging if you are seeing a child who is 6 months overdue for her well
visit, particularly if she is brought in 1 h late by her mother. In such
an instance we might go out of our way to let the mother know how
important it is that she has brought her daughter in to catch up on her
immunizations. This would be unconditional positive regard, as
opposed to showing frustration and scolding the mother for this delay.
Similarly, a 30-year-old, two-packs-per-day smoker can be applauded
for having cut down to half a pack over the past week. In fact, we can
find something positive in the behaviors of everyone we see.

It is not always easy to put unconditional positive regard into prac-
tice. According to Dr. Adrienne Williams, Director of Behavioral
Science in the Department of Family and Community Medicine at the
University of Maryland School of Medicine:

Many clinicians try to keep things positive by balancing negative
statements with something positive, such as "You really need to do

R. Colgan, *Advice to the Healer: On the Art of Caring*,
DOI 10.1007/978-1-4614-5170-9_8,
© Springer Science+Business Media, LLC 2013

much better, but I know you tried hard." However, this is not unconditional positive regard, and patients will generally only attend to the negative part of the sentence ("you really need to do much better") and feel judged, chastised, or deflated.

Unconditional positive regard uses only the positive part of the sentence which supports the patient, and avoids the demoralization, defensiveness, or loss of motivation that negative statements can trigger. So the clinician might say "You tried really hard!" and then offer support that moves the patient forward, such as "This is really difficult to do, and each time you try you get closer to accomplishing your goal". [Personal Communication with Dr. A. Williams]

We can practice unconditional positive regard in our relationship with each patient despite not being a psychiatrist, psychologist, or licensed clinical social worker.

A healer will see the technique of unconditional positive regard as an opportunity to strengthen the clinician–patient relationship. You will also improve your patient's self-image and compliance. This is a "win-win" situation!

We may not be professional counselors, but we are professionals who counsel. Rogers offered four specific techniques which can help clinicians who are not trained therapists build therapeutic relationships with their patients [1].

The first is by showing warmth and responsiveness. This allows for better rapport and, in turn, leads to a deeper emotional relationship. Looking your patients in the eye and greeting them with a smile shows warmth. Being able to see a patient who has an urgent problem and returning calls promptly demonstrates respect and sensitivity to his or her needs, as well as your responsiveness.

The second quality of a therapeutic relationship is permissiveness in regard to expression of feeling. Permissiveness as used here means not being judgmental or rigid, particularly if the patient's opinion or behaviors run contrary to our own. You may not agree with your patients' political views, lifestyle, or religious beliefs. A doctor recently made national news for posting a sign on his office door telling patients who voted for President Barack Obama to seek care elsewhere, as he considered the President's national health care overhaul to be bad medicine. This may be viewed by some as an example of not being permissive. Everyone we serve is deserving of our respect.

Thirdly, we should understand the therapeutic limits of each visit with a patient. Time is one example of a limit. If patients do arrive late and you are unable to work them into your schedule (because you are seeing other patients who arrived on time), patients should not be free to control your schedule. If you are able to attend to the patient properly in the amount of time you have, that is fine, but it is also acceptable to explain to him or her that you are not able to address the complaint at this time. You might add that you do not want to rush and do a suboptimal job. You can prevent this from happening by determining "all" of their goals at the beginning. Ask them what they would like to discuss today, and follow-up with any specific goals you have: "I see that your blood pressure is very high. I want to be sure we address this as well."

The fourth characteristic of Rogers' helpful therapeutic relationship is freedom from any type of pressure or coercion. This does not necessarily apply to all clinical situations, as I think there are times when appropriate pressure coupled with informed consent is appropriate. A patient who is resistant to going to the emergency room for atrial fibrillation or chest pain, for example, must be told in clear terms why such a strong recommendation is being made. Rogers' advice could best be applied to a situation like one that arose with a resident I worked with who considered herself a sort of fitness guru. She frequently recommended to patients that they drink eight glasses of water every day and take vitamins. I brought to her attention that I could not find evidence-based medical literature to support her opinion. Neither could she. She is entitled to her opinion, but Rogers might say we should not pressure our patients into doing what we want them to do.

Nonprofessionally trained therapists serving as counselors, you may ask? Sure, we do it all the time. Drs. Marian Stuart and Joseph Lieberman have written extensively how to do just that in their book *The Fifteen Minute Hour: Therapeutic Talk in Primary Care*. In this book, and in other teaching tools, they note the goals of 15-min therapy are: (1) preventing dire consequences; (2) reestablishing premorbid level of functioning; (3) expanding behavioral repertoire; and (4) enhancing patients' self-esteem. The authors offer the BATHE technique as a useful tool to every clinician [2]. "How to Bathe your patients as you SOAP them" follows:

How to BATHE Your Patients as You SOAP Them

*B*ackground: "What is going on in your life?"
*A*ffect/Feeling: "How are you feeling about that?"
*T*rouble: "What troubles you the most?"
*H*andling: "How are you handling that?"
*E*mpathy: "That must be must be very difficult."

The authors urge the adoption of therapeutic skills using a new paradigm. This paradigm recognizes that: (1) We constantly tell ourselves, as well as others, stories; (2) These stories create our reality and affect our experience; (3) The stories reflect our view of who we are; and (4) These stories determine what we are capable of doing. The authors point out that psychotherapy means editing the story. First, the story must be heard. Second, the story must be reflected back with empathy and third, the limits offered by the patient must be challenged. Patients may impose their own challenging limits as when they utter words such as *can't, must, should,* and *it's impossible.* Strategies offered for helping patients include (1) Focusing on options: Don't tell your patients what they should do, but ask them "what are your options?" (2) Looking at consequences: ask your patient: "what's the worst thing that could happen if you did this?" or "the best scenario if you chose that... what are the likelihoods of each?" (3) Applying the tincture of time: pointing out that things will change if you just hang in there and (4) Choosing not to choose: help your patients understand that they are in control. Should someone give them an ultimatum, e.g., "I am going to leave you unless...." Point out that by not accepting this ultimatum they are in control. The other person will have to decide what to do if you choose not to participate in the challenge.

The authors go on to describe four options to point out in a bad situation: leave it, change it, accept it, and reframe it. By putting the patients in control, we focus on their strengths, delineate responsibility for behavior, and aim for small wins. As clinicians who counsel, we can remind our patients that the past is gone, the future is not here, and we can only act/feel in the here and now.

The preceding tips on the 15-min therapeutic hour are offered to gain your interest in pursuing these and other therapeutic techniques. I am not suggesting that by merely reading the above paragraphs you are ready to provide comprehensive therapy. On the contrary, there is a difference between incorporating therapeutic skills in your clinical encounters and providing therapy. Readers wanting to learn more about how to better their skills in providing counseling within the context of our current profession are urged to review the suggested reading section at the end of this chapter.

Rogers tells us that we all want and need love and acceptance. This can be shown to our patients by showing them unconditional positive regard. Contemporary clinicians Stuart and Lieberman would add that our ability to listen and the words we chose to respond with are one of the most valuable and underused tools a healer has.

Choosing Good Practice

It's smart to avoid malpractice. It's smarter to choose good practice. Good doctors, young and old, practicing good medicine, charting good medical records still get sued. So how can you avoid this? In this section we will give you some tips on how to keep the threat of a lawsuit to a minimum.[1]

Definition of Malpractice

Medical malpractice suits fall under the categorization of personal injury or tort law, of which there are three different classifications: negligence, strict liability, and intentional torts. These causes of action are civil (not criminal) and address liability and the nature and extent of damages. Malpractice suits arise when a patient alleges negligence committed by a professional health care provider. To prove negligence, a court must find that the health care provider deviated from the standard of care deemed reasonable by those with similar training and experience, under similar circumstances, and that this breach in their performance of duties caused harm or injury to a patient. Usually other doctors are called to testify as expert witnesses

---

[1]Originally published in a modified format in Maryland Family Doctor, Winter 2009 and authored by Colgan, Richard; Colgan, Kathleen, and Farley, Robert.

and give their opinion as to whether a health care provider's actions fell below the accepted standard of care and to testify as to what a competent physician would have done under the same or similar circumstances. Thus, the standard for malpractice is set by the medical profession itself, by its own practices and customs.

Common Lawsuits

Before discussing some common malpractice situations, it should be emphasized that the best practices in the physician–patient relationship entail good communication with the patient, and where appropriate (and with the patient's permission) his or her family. Being sure that your patient understands what you do is critical. At times having that understanding written down and signed is even better. All of us have made mistakes, and most physicians will tell you that with each patient a "credit account" exists whereupon errors or withdrawals are tallied compared with the more common "good doctoring" deposits. The truth is that most patients respect their physicians and few bring malpractice suits. So while it is important that you practice good medicine and document well, the most important reason why a patient does *not* bring a suit against a doctor is his or her interpretation of a satisfactory physician–patient relationship that has developed, both over time and especially around the time of the alleged transgression.

Leading the list of common medical malpractice suits are those cases under the heading of undiagnosed or late diagnosis of a catastrophe that ended in either significant morbidity or mortality for the patient. Both perceived and real errors can lead to a claim of medical malpractice.

Missed Myocardial Ischemia

A common failure is neglecting to appreciate that ischemia can present with epigastric pain, dyspnea, or other atypical symptoms. Similarly, ordering an electrocardiogram only to conclude that your patient does not have a myocardial infarction because the electrocardiogram appears normal is an error. The teaching pearl is: If you think that someone may be having acute coronary syndrome based on the history, there are a few particular things on the physical exam or electrocardiogram which may likely mitigate that risk. This is where clinical judgment comes in. The risk of myocardial infarction is higher if there is a gallop, hypotension, or pain radiating to both arms, and less if the pain is pleuritic and reproducible by palpating the chest wall.

Missed Acute Abdomen

The classical presentation of acute appendicitis is well known; however, patients often present in a nonclassical fashion. Two elements in the typical history of appendicitis are the presence of anorexia and the determination that the patients' pain, or whatever specific description of "dis–ease" they may use, is constant. One of the best predictors that your patients may be suffering from appendicitis is if the pain is reported (you may have to ask them) to have moved from the periumbilical area to the right lower quadrant. Other subtle findings for nonclassical appendicitis are the presence of Dunfy's sign: abdominal pain with coughing; Rovsing's sign: right lower quadrant pain with palpation of the left lower quadrant; Iliopsoas test: abdominal pain with extension of the right leg against resistance; and jar tenderness: guarding or pain with sudden movements such as bumping the examining table, jumping in place, or hitting the patient's heel.

Failing to Inform Your Patients That They Are at High Risk

Another general category of malpractice risk is failure to explain to the patient or his or her family just how sick the patient is. This is particularly true when you have not yet had the time to develop a longitudinal relationship with your patient. This occurs commonly in instances when you see a new patient that you immediately identify as being very sick or with a high likelihood of an impending catastrophe. In situations like this it may be appropriate to "hang crepe paper[2]," i.e., to explain to the patient and family that your assessment concludes that he or she may be suffering from a very serious condition, and that if this is indeed the true diagnosis, it entails a high risk of further morbidity or mortality. Unfortunately such life-threatening illnesses do occur, and it is the physician's responsibility to inform the patients that they have, for example, lung cancer, pancreatic cancer, or similar conditions where the life expectancy may be as little as 6 months. Another example is that of a new patient who presents to you with New York Heart Association Class 4 congestive heart failure, which also carries a high risk of death.[2]

What Your Defense Attorney Wants You to Know

Just because a patient files a lawsuit against you does not mean that it possesses legal or factual merit. The task for the practitioner is learning how to best avoid becoming a malpractice defendant in the first place and, if you *are* sued, to know what you can do to most effectively assist your defense team (your attorney and malpractice carrier) in representing you.

Many malpractice suits are filed because a patient or his or her family is surprised by the result(s) of a course of treatment or intervention. Often this is because of a perceived incorrect or "missed" diagnosis or is a consequence of a family's frustration with a "bad outcome." If patients and their families are able to understand the proposed treatment or intervention in the context of the patient's pre-existing medical condition(s), as well as realize the reality of the less-than-perfect state of medicine—that an outcome cannot be guaranteed or controlled—then there is less "surprise" experienced if something bad happens to the patient. It therefore follows that open and frank discussions with the patient and family are paramount in diminishing the surprise of a bad outcome and hopefully quelling the need for a lawsuit.

By far, the most significant "weapon" in your malpractice defense arsenal is the patient's medical chart and your own proper charting in the records. For a malpractice case to survive preliminary legal

---

[2]The term "hanging crepe paper" draws from an old custom of pinning black paper around the home's parlor entrance when the death of its inhabitant was perceived to be imminent.

challenge, the patient's attorney must secure an independent review of the medical records by another health care provider. This person is ultimately required to opine, based on review of the records, that there has or has not been a deviation from applicable standards of care. So, the patient's medical record is both your "sword and shield" as its review might result in the failure of the patient to secure the requisite reviewer's critical opinion and moreover, if suit follows through, the record becomes the foundation of your defense to the alleged negligence. It is imperative that you do your reasonable best to chart clearly, accurately, and in a timely manner. However, that does not mean writing a novel for each patient encounter. Rather, note the time of your hospital chart entries as well as when exactly you saw the patient in an effective manner so that a timeline of your patient encounters can be re-created after the fact. Enter a brief summary of discussions you have with the patient, family, and other providers that are of significance to the patient's care (such as passing of orders of a specific nature to a consultant). Write a brief sentence or two of your reasoning for recommending a certain treatment, especially when there may be some disagreement as to its efficacy. Make your charts thorough but concise, keeping in mind that if a suit comes around, the properly documented patient chart is your best defense against any malpractice allegations.

If you are served with a lawsuit, you should first preserve the integrity of the patient's medical record. Ensure that the record is in a safe place to begin with (that is, do not "lose or misplace it"). Most importantly, under no circumstances should you endeavor to edit, change, delete, or seek to complete or embellish any of the past entries you or any other individual has made in the patient's medical record! When—not if—discovered, this will result in dire consequences for you and your medical career. If you were to make edits or alterations to the medical record, you should clearly indicate that you are looking to amend the record, reasons for the changes, and the date/time that the changes are made.

Next, you must notify your malpractice insurance carrier of the lawsuit. Remember, even before you have been served with court papers, the patient has already found a lawyer who has investigated the case and deemed it significant enough to follow through with a suit. Therefore, there should be little delay in this notification. You want the carrier to get up to speed as soon as possible in preparing the defense of your case, which includes opening a case file and securing defense counsel on your behalf. Avoid the understandable instinct to speak to others about the fact of this lawsuit or the specifics of your care and treatment of the patient-plaintiff other than representatives of your insurance carrier and your attorney's office. Loose lips sink ships. When speaking to your representatives, speak truthfully, openly, and candidly about the facts of the case and the allegations as you understand them. The defense team will best be able to represent and defend your interests if you tell the truth, even if the truth is "bad, negligent, or ugly."

Work with your malpractice carrier and your defense counsel in developing your theory of defense and offering assistance on the medical aspect of the case. This team truly has the successful defense of your interests as their primary objective. Consider engaging in the academic exercise of the reasons that medically and factually your care, management, and treatment met the applicable standards of care and did not cause the patient's alleged injury. By doing so, you will have taken the important first step in developing the defense theory for your case. The defense of a malpractice lawsuit is truly a team effort in which you are a significant contributor! Not only that, but you have the most at stake.

Finally, your attorney will keep you advised of the process of the litigation, answer your questions, and counsel you throughout. He or she is your advocate and you should not hesitate to ask him or her questions as to the proposed strategy in defending you, as well as the consequences of any feasible outcome.

While medical errors may be inevitable, you can choose to lessen your risk of being served with a malpractice suit. Being aware of the type of clinical scenarios which are more commonly the reason for filing suits, establishing good rapport with your patients, including a frank discussion about their conditions, and contacting your malpractice carrier's legal team as soon as you are concerned about an incident are absolutely critical. The litigation process is dynamic, so maintaining an open line of communication with defense is a must. And, you will survive!

References

1. Rogers C, Kramer Peter D. On becoming a person: a therapist's view of psychotherapy. Boston, MA: Mariner Books; 1995.
2. Stuart MR, Lieberman JA, Rakel RE. The fifteen minute hour: therapeutic talk in primary care. 4th ed. Oxford and New York: Radcliffe Publishing; 2008.

Clinicians as Counselors

Stuart MR, Lieberman JA, Rakel RE. The fifteen minute hour: therapeutic talk in primary care. 4th ed. Oxford and New York: Radcliffe Publishing; 2008.

Rogers C, Kramer Peter D. On becoming a person: a therapist's view of psychotherapy. Boston, MA: Mariner Books; 1995.

Rogers CR. Client-centered therapy: it's current practice, implications, and theory, Constable, 1995. http://15minutehour.com. Accessed 27 May 2012.

Chapter 9
A Doctor's Journal

Searching for the True Poetry of Life

Here's the good news: Almost every one of you, once you are a licensed professional or professionally acknowledged healer in service to mankind, will live relatively comfortable lives. At least you will unlikely suffer from the structural violence (lack of food, water, shelter and health care) described by Farmer. As highly educated, respected members of your community, you will spend your working days using your training to help others. What a fulfilling way to make a living! The downside is that you are entering into, or are currently working in a vocation that requires you to work extremely hard, commit to long hours and rough days, and deal with many emotionally stressful situations. There will be times when you wonder if it was all worth it. You will see friends that earn more money than you, who perhaps seem to experience fewer difficulties in their occupations. You will have bad days when you simply wonder why you got into the field. Osler has a suggestion on how you can stay enthusiastic when things look dark:

> "Nothing will sustain you more potently than the power to recognize in your humdrum routine, as perhaps it may be thought, the true poetry of life—the poetry of the commonplace, of the ordinary man, of the plain, toil-worn woman, with their loves and their joys, their sorrows and their griefs" [1].

I add that it is even better to write it down. Healers are in a great position to begin keeping or maintaining a diary, journal, or blog in which memorable stories are saved. I urge you to write down some of these more memorable stories and look back on them often.

R. Colgan, *Advice to the Healer: On the Art of Caring*,
DOI 10.1007/978-1-4614-5170-9_9,
© Springer Science+Business Media, LLC 2013

Reading these stories years later, as your wisdom increases and your beliefs evolve, will sustain you.

The American poet and general practitioner William Carlos Williams, (1883–1963) "worked harder at being a writer than he did at being a physician," wrote the biographer Linda Wagner-Martin [2]. Williams felt that being a practitioner of medicine helped him become a better writer. I admit to being inspired by William's *Doctor Stories*, a wonderful collection of tales that I highly recommend since it illustrates what one practitioner can create by simply putting his or her own stories down on paper. You shouldn't worry if you do not see yourself as the same caliber of writer as Williams. That's not the point. Rather, each one of us has at least one story which could be published if crafted properly. For assistance in moving forward I recommend Robert B. Taylor's *Medical Writing*, second edition, on this subject.

I hope reading these entries will encourage you to begin your own collection of writings. As memorable events occur, you will discover that they grow dim over time and are eventually forgotten. Surely, looking back on what you considered to be significant experiences throughout the years will bring you back—not only to those events themselves, but to that time and place, to the life events surrounding you then. These memories are true treasures. They perk you up after depressing or difficult days. They ground you when you feel overwhelmed. They remind you why you became a healer and hopefully inspire you to continue your extraordinary work.

Recollections

Although many situations in medicine are often difficult, some of the most poetic moments we encounter in practice are incredibly positive, uplifting, or just plain funny. What follows are a few entries from a journal I started years ago, when I first began private practice.

Gregory B. is an adorable 3-year-old boy whose mother brought him in to see me for a number of complaints. He's been suffering from a cough along with some nasal discharge, a bellyache, and some assorted bodily pains, among many other issues. As his mother listed concern after concern, I directed the interview to the preschooler himself. I asked Gregory, "What bothers you the most?" His eyes opened wide as he immediately thought of his answer. "Fire... and snakes in the mud!" he chirped. His mother explained that in fact last night he had experienced a nightmare with those exact images, and to that extent she felt this response was accurate.

Children definitely describe symptoms differently than adults. Stephanie B. is a 7-year-old who was experiencing some gastrointestinal distress. She described this innocently as, "It feels like a feather in my throat... like birds taking a bath in my stomach."

I met a 6-year-old boy, sitting on the examining table looking annoyed. He had a different chief complaint than what was described in the nurse's note. I asked the boy what bothered him the most, other than the reported "cough." He looked once towards his parents, who were sitting to his left and said, "When I am trying to talk and people, like these two here, interrupt me." When I asked him if anything else bothered him, he said, "Yeah, when I am trying to watch TV and people stand in front of it."

A smartly dressed, well-spoken gentleman saw me at the office with the chief complaint of a sore throat. From the start of the visit, it was clear that he wanted to provide me a very specific and detailed description of his condition. During the course of the interview, he pointed to the normal "punching bag structure" found dangling from posterior aspect of his soft palate (known medically as the uvula). He cited that what bothered him most was his "vulva." I immediately asked him to repeat his answer, as I was not sure I heard him correctly. "I saw that my vulva was swollen," he said. I now faced a dilemma: Should I correct him on the proper use of the word "uvula?" Should I ruin this humor for all doctors down the road who might otherwise hear his mistake? I won't tell you my decision.

Margaret R. is a proper 68-year-old lady from London, England. I have taken care of her for many years, and over this time we have enjoyed many laughs together. During a routine sigmoidoscopic exam, I asked her if she would like to have a look inside, as I have asked all of my other patients in the past when performing this exam. This would be accomplished by turning the scope so she too could look through the eyepiece, I explained. She replied, "That would be quite lovely." As she peered through the scope, this cheerful British woman exclaimed, "This is quite marvelous! It rather looks like the planets doesn't it?"

"I have never thought of it that way before," I replied. "But if you had to think of any one planet that it looks like, you'd have to say it looks like Uranus." The nurse bumped into the surgical tray, instruments fell to the floor, and I began to think that perhaps I had gone too far in being familiar in attempt to joke around with my patient. Thoughts of calls to the Board of Physicians by my patient or the surgical nurse began to enter my mind.

I didn't see this patient again for a year, which convinced me that indeed I had offended her and prompted her to seek care elsewhere. When she did return a year later I greeted her with a warm hello and told her that I thought she had fired me because of the comment I made during our last visit. "What? No, I am sorry," she said. "I don't remember that." As it turned out, she moved back to England to care for a sick relative and had not given the off-colored joke a second thought. She and I were both happy to continue our special physician–patient relationship.

Poems from Private Practice

Searching for the poetry of life is not merely another checkbox to be completed after each patient visit; it does not fall in line right after documenting vital signs and recording the review of systems. Rather, this adage encourages us to be cognizant of the human side of our patients. Or, as one doctor once described to me, "Acknowledge the patient's underside, their soft belly side, the side they do not show the rest of society." One of the many privileges of being a healer is that patients are willing to share this side with us. I am astounded at how often I think I know a patient only to later learn more about this person's "poetry of life." It also reminds me why I love medicine so much. What follows are some longer poems, each of which has important life lessons we all can learn from if we focus on each patient.

He Apologized, Twice

One night while working late at the health center in the middle of one of the worst downpours I had ever witnessed, out of the corner of my eye I caught sight of a man lumbering into our waiting room soaking wet. I judged him to be no more than 30 years old, but he walked slowly with the aid of two mid-thigh-high wooden walking sticks. This was towards the end of a 12-h day seeing patients in our inner city academic primary care clinic—I remember I was longing to go home.

At nearly ten 'til seven, the medical assistant asked me if I wanted my 6 p.m. patient, who had only just arrived, to reschedule. Not knowing it was the same man I had seen earlier, I said, "No, I'll see him." This was how I met Michael.

When I walked into the examining room, I was initially intrigued by Michael's appearance. It was only later that I became aware of his humanity. What was most striking about him was his head of tangled hair. It was neither well combed nor recently washed and foretold what I might see while looking over the man. When we did make eye contact, I remember thinking how strikingly innocent and needful he was.

Michael's coat was as old and worn as the library book he was reading, the title of which surprised me. In his hand he held an eso-teric philosophy textbook that I imagined had not been checked out by anyone for many years. I felt bad for having noticed several old and new stains on his shirt and was slightly embarrassed to be so obviously better dressed than he was. He did not have control of his body, and he would occasionally twist this way and that. His mouth struggled when he spoke. He had difficulty holding his body still or making it do simple things like laying down his book, which he did when I entered the exam room.

"I'm sorry I was late," he said, before I had the chance to intro-duce myself. Suddenly filled with curiosity, I wanted to know more about him. I was surprised to learn that his parents, whom I used to take care of when I practiced elsewhere, had referred Michael to me. I recalled them, a silver-haired couple sitting in a different room in another city 5 years earlier, telling me how they were looking forward to moving to a warmer climate in California. They spoke in passing of their only son, Michael, who lived in the city where I now worked and who had been born with a neuromuscular disorder. Although they expressed some concern about moving away, they exhibited a calmness about them that I assumed was the reward for decades of successful parenting. They seemed to be confident he would do well. "Would you be his doctor?" they asked upon learning that I, too, was leaving to practice in the same city.

Checking Michael's records, I learned that he had sought my help once before but was seen by another physician in my absence. A year earlier, a potentially life-threatening infection prompted his direct admission to our hospital, after which he underwent emergency surgery. Several months later, he was discharged from a rehabilitation unit to return home and care for himself again. So many questions ran through my head during the first few minutes of our encounter. Did his parents come to see him? Did he have friends to visit him? Did his neighbors watch out for him? Would he be missed at the mailbox if something happened and he didn't show? I was struck then with his seemingly lonely independence.

The purpose of tonight's visit was for a refill of an antidepressant medication. We talked about the book he was reading. He sought my opinion as to whether or not he would be able to resume a search for employment once again. Throughout the visit I was struck by how different he looked from the man I saw in the waiting room and how accommodating his behavior was to me, the doctor, the one he needed right now to get a refill for an expensive pill that helped treat his mental illness. How did he afford this medication on a disability income? After finding samples in our drug closet of what he needed, we worked out a plan for a follow-up visit. Standing up from the stool (a doctor's cue that the visit is over), I extended my hand and told Michael I looked forward to seeing him again. Still apologetic, he attempted to close the visit by whispering once again, "I'm sorry I was late." Patients have apologized to me before for this very reason, and often I accept their apology and continue my day without giving it a second thought. Sensing there was more he wanted to say I asked, "Why were you late, Michael?" I was not prepared for his answer.

I learned that Michael relied on public transportation. This was the reason he didn't move with his parents; the bus system where they live is nowhere near as good as the one in our city. He told me that night he had taken the No. 7 bus from his apartment across town to the closest stop near our health center. He walked the remaining 12 blocks from the bus stop, in heavy rain, with the aid of his two wooden walking sticks. I asked how long it had taken him to make this trek down the rainy street and, without expression, he replied, "About 20 minutes." I was shocked. This must have been excruciatingly difficult for a person in his physical condition.

At the 1996 Democratic National Convention, Christopher Reeve, the actor who suffered a grave spinal cord injury, gave an unforgettable speech. Some of what he said reminded me of Michael and his family. Mr. Reeve mesmerized his audience as he sat tightly belted in his wheelchair, saying:

> "Over the last few years we've heard a lot about something called family values. And like many of you I've struggled to figure out what that means. But since my accident I've found a definition that seems to make sense. I think it means we're all family, and that we all have values. And if that is true, if America really is family, then we have to recognize that much of our family is hurting" [3].

These thoughts filled my mind as I looked at Michael. If Michael was hurting that night, he didn't complain to me, his physician. How could he not have been hurting after such a difficult struggle to get here? The image of this civil, soft-spoken, disabled man is perhaps familiar to many of us. He may have been like many men we see on a city street corner, an image that cues us to turn the other way. If our eyes meet, we are forced to face something painful we would rather ignore.

The fact that a member of our family felt the need to apologize twice for the slight inconvenience he had caused me has to touch your heart. Michael's story represents but one of many more which go unnoticed, and that should make us weep. As medical practitioners, we have been given a special opportunity, a privilege, to share in an intimate and helpful relationship with patients from our cultures, as well as those from completely different backgrounds. In our fast-paced practices, it is easy to get consumed by busy days and tight schedules. Further, the increasing dominance of technology in medical practice creates an atmosphere that makes it easy to trivialize the need and value of the healer's art.

What can we—as healers—take away from Michael's story? One lesson may be that cultural diversity also includes those who are different then us, aside from ethnicity, socioeconomic class, or religion. Those who live with disabilities are outside of my culture. Perhaps we need to remind ourselves to listen more actively so that we may hear our patients and tap into what makes them unique individuals.

If we do not look outside our culture, we may miss meeting other members of our human family. Most importantly, if we overlook the opportunity to extend our hand to someone in need, we will ultimately be the ones that find ourselves alone and unfulfilled.

Michael never returned to see me for his follow-up visit. Two years after our initial encounter, I found him waiting in another exam room on another doctor's schedule. I asked if it would be alright if I saw him and he agreed. He told me that since we last met he had been diagnosed with a more serious mental illness and was hospitalized for several months. He was still looking for a job and still loved to read. I did my best to reconnect with Michael and urged him to come back and see me, so that I could be his regular doctor. He said he would.

When he didn't keep his follow-up visit, I called Michael's home repeatedly. There was never an answer, and I continue to be unable to reach him. It has been 10 years.

From this experience with Michael, I have changed my practice for the better. Now, if a patient arrives late, I think twice about asking him or her to reschedule and try to consider each individual's story.

A Modern Family

[(Richard Colgan, Caitlin Iafolla Zaner) Reproduced with permission from JAMA, A Piece of My Mind November 24, 2010-Vol 304, No.20].

I first met Joe on the 13th floor of an inner-city hospital. He was lying comfortably in his hospital bed, granted refuge as an unassigned medical admission for chest pain the night before by the inpatient team. Joe was a 73-year-old white man with uncombed hair, bushy eyebrows, and a severely stooped posture noticeable even as he sat upright in the bed. He had a gravelly voice—from years of smoking, I soon learned. On the chair beside him were his clothes, which were worn well beyond their life expectancy. Joe looked like someone who had worked hard all his life and appeared much older than his actual age. Aside from his appearance, I was struck by the tattered text by his bedside. It was an old edition of Age of Enlightenment, with "Enoch Pratt Library" stamped on the first page.

While taking his history and performing a physical examination, I noticed that Joe spoke brusquely with many facial twitches and gross motor disturbances. He did not use many big words. I asked him politely about his book to which he replied, oddly, "Oh, you know. I enjoy reading works of philosophy, particularly about Erasmus and the Reformation." I had heard of Erasmus before, but was not very familiar with his history or theories. Joe knew all about this subject. He told me that he loved to read. I asked him about the last book he read. "Mein Kampf," he replied. I asked him what he read before this, and he answered, "The Rise and Fall of the Third Reich." I wondered to myself, who is this guy? As it turned out, he wasn't a Nazi at all but absolutely loved all types of military history. His most recent reads had focused on the world wars. Joe's favorite was the 1895 war novel *The Red Badge of Courage* by Stephen Crane. Joe continued, "But what I am really looking for, Doc, is a book about World War II by an American author—not a British author—but an American author." Given my first impression of Joe, I was surprised to learn of his scholarly pursuits.

Joe was born and raised on the east side of Baltimore and had made it through seventh grade. When I asked him why he didn't go further in school, he said, "I quit school the day my father died, so I could go to work at a warehouse to help support my mother." He had always loved reading and learning and tried his best to make time for these activities. At the age of 21, he married. It was also at this time that he developed schizophrenia. Unfortunately this factor, as he explained it, was likely in part why his marriage failed after only 2 months and resulted in no children. That same year Joe was admitted to a state psychiatric hospital, followed by another stay at a different state hospital. These were the first of what were many psychiatric admissions; longer and longer each time and which ultimately became a 30-year period of institutionalization. His twisted facial expressions and thrashing body movements were caused by the cumulative adverse effects of years of powerful antipsychotic medications, which only dampened his disturbing thoughts and the obtrusive voices he experienced. Despite all this, Joe was beloved by the hospital staff, where he held the reputation as an exemplary patient. Eventually he earned the privileges to work as an employee, supervising others in the boiler room. The institution became his home. In 1981, President Ronald Reagan rescinded the Mental Health Systems Act of 1980, which resulted in reduced federal funding to community mental health centers. Many patients, who were no longer thought to be a threat to themselves or to others, were released from intensive psychiatric care. This included Joe. After leaving the facility, Joe was offered and accepted a job to continue working at the hospital as a paid employee, with room and board included. Inexplicably, after a year of compensated service, he left.

For years after his departure from psychiatric institutionalization, Joe was dutifully cared for by Miss Elsie, a 60-year-old African American woman. Elsie was herself no stranger to difficult times. She had married twice during her life; both marriages ended in divorce from abusive husbands. For more than 25 years she worked long hours as a correctional officer. After retirement from this career, she opened up an adult care service in her two-story four-bedroom home in a working-class suburb of Baltimore. Elsie was contacted in 2004 by an admiring social worker from a local hospital, who asked if she would accept a new client under her care. She was told this gentleman had resided in substandard housing under horrible conditions—essentially in a room that was little more than a mattress on a basement floor and virtually void of human contact. This is how Joe first met Miss Elsie, a stranger who would walk beside him for the rest of his life.

Joe had neither living relatives nor close friends. He often spent his time alone. On a weekly basis, Joe took the local bus to the Enoch Pratt Library, where he would read for hours. On a good day he would walk away with free books in hand. "I can't believe they give these things away!" he excitedly told me. His prized collection comprised a nine-book series by Zane Grey stamped "Not for Resale/This Is a Free Book." Other favorites were Theodore H. White's *In Search of History, The Outline of History* by H. G. Wells, and *Words That Made American History* by Current and Garraty. Reading and extensive volunteer work helped keep his inner voices away. He was well known for his charitable services at the same inner-city hospital I met him. He worked for years, wearing a blue smock as he pushed patients in wheelchairs to their destinations around the wards. Miss Elsie noted that Joe had no close friends, recalling, "His friends were all those who he saw… everywhere he went."

But Joe's tranquil life would quickly change. A workup for escalating chest pain revealed a tumor noted on CT scan. I asked Joe to come to the office to discuss this, which he did with a book in hand and Miss Elsie by his side. He would need a biopsy, I explained to the two of them, which took place several days later. Joe entertained the staff in interventional radiology while recovering from the outpatient procedure. He allowed eight Introduction to Clinical Medicine students to ask him questions about his background and to examine him. His biopsy showed "many hypermitotic cells." "It's adenocarcinoma," explained the attending pathologist to the students and me as we sat around a spider-like microscope with 16 heads in the basement of the hospital. Once the anesthesia wore off, Elsie took him home. Despite only 2 months of aggressive chemotherapy, Joe was thought to no longer be a candidate for cure or betterment and returned home for hospice care.

Joe continued to reside with Miss Elsie in her home. At our last home visit, my group of medical students and I were able to see the love and care that Elsie showed him—the difference she had made for this man. One student stood crying softly to herself behind Joe, as he sat in his recliner and tried to reassure us that he was in no pain. She told me that she had never been around someone who was so close to death. Still seated, Joe waved good-bye to us as we left that day with the directive he always gave at the end of each visit: "Take care of yourself now." Just 1 week later, on a Saturday morning, I received an unexpected telephone call from Miss Elsie. "He's gone," she somberly informed me. "Joe. I found him dead this morning when I went into his room."

Joe and Elsie certainly were a nontraditional family. They were two strangers brought together by difficult circumstances and who developed a caring and supportive relationship. She not only provided him with shelter, food, and his basic necessities but showed him kindness, respect, friendship, and love. Joe reciprocated her dedication by giving Elsie someone to listen to and a helper around the house who often tried to complete chores despite his declining health. He frequently went out of his way to compliment and recognize her for all that she did for him. "You deserve better than this," he often told her.

Joe taught us humility, perseverance, and grace. His relationship with his caregiver illustrates the notion that not all families are alike, that they cannot easily be defined. Further, that by recognizing and supporting these nontraditional family relationships, physicians are better able to understand their patients and thus provide more individual and humanistic health care. When asked of Joe now, Miss Elsie is thankful and reflects, "He gives me the strength to keep on going."

Before he died, Joe told me how much he enjoyed the two American-authored World War II books I sent him. Elsie suggested to Joe that upon his death he allow her to make a trip to Harpers Ferry, Virginia, to spread his ashes over a military battlefield. He liked the idea. However, she learned after his death that because she was not next of kin, nor had any recognized legal relationship to Joe, she would not be able to receive his ashes. Perhaps there was some consolation in knowing that she was able to honor his other dying wish. Miss Elsie was successful in helping Joe complete the necessary paperwork so that he could donate his body to the state anatomy board, located next door to the hospital where he had volunteered his services for years.

A Meaningful Life

The door was open to the exam room and inside I saw a 6′2 inch tall white man pacing back and forth. I was struck by the great difficulty he had in speaking and breathing. His face was covered with sweat. His mouth contorted like a Cheshire cat as he spoke in short jerking cadences. I immediately wanted to know more about him.

His name was Ted, and he told me he was there for a check on his blood pressure. He explained that the reason why he thrust his left arm into the air repeatedly as he spoke in loud grunts was because it helped him speak more clearly. He knew people find it hard to understand him. Ted had involuntary eye blinking and acted like his neck muscles were too tight.

I also learned that he had a long history of not taking his psychiatric pills because of a great distrust of psychiatric medications in general. His medical record listed paranoid schizophrenia, depression, obsessive-compulsive disorder, and tardive dyskinesia as his problems. As he left the office he asked me, "Have they found a cure for tardive dyskinesia yet?" I told him I didn't think so, but I'd try to see if there was anything new in the literature.

Over the course of several visits I came to learn that Ted wasn't always like this.

With great difficulty in expressing himself, Ted told me of graduating from high school with a B average and going to college where he graduated (with honors) in history. He liked volunteering and, after helping high school dropouts get their GED, he went on to earn two Masters Degrees, including a Masters of Social Work. He worked as a social worker for several years until his life began to spin out of control.

Several years later, while living largely out of his car, he was arrested for theft, trespassing, assault and battery, and malicious destruction of property after an angry outburst while trying to pay a late charge for oversleeping in a hotel. He spent 40 days in a county detention center and had his car impounded. This was followed by another detention center stay after being charged with threatening a judge over the phone. "I was just angry and blew off steam," he explained to me. Ted's father influenced the judge to find him not guilty by reason of insanity, and this was followed by his first commitment at a state psychiatric hospital. He was awarded a conditional release for 3 years as long as he took all of his prescribed medications, which included powerful antipsychotics like thorazine. This pattern of not taking his oral psychiatric medications would continue throughout his life.

Ted continued to go in and out different group homes, interrupted by psychiatric institutionalizations during which he was ordered to take major tranquilizers. In an effort to help him, his doctors escalated his therapy to monthly injections of fluphenazine because of his history of refusing oral medications and noncompliance. This led to Ted acquiring tardive dyskinesia (TD), a disorder he was at risk for by virtue of having a prolonged exposure to antipsychotics—especially a depot high potency first-generation agent and his older age. Neuroleptics like fluphenazine not only display increased liability to cause TD but can also paradoxically mask TD so that involuntary movements are not evident until discontinuation of the drug, known as "withdrawal-emergent dyskinesias".

Ted disputes that he suffers from schizophrenia. "I don't believe this. I decompensate when something is stolen or lost, or I am violated. I get agitated and depressed." He notes that he's never heard voices, never had suicidal or homicidal ideation and adds "no gambling, drinking, drugs, or cigarettes."

Ted's tragedies would not be behind him. His father died of a heart attack when Ted was 35 years old, yet fortunately his mother, whom he deeply loved, continued to support and care for him. "She was an extremely good mother." He soon found pleasure in nothing more than when he was with her. With saliva involuntarily falling from the left side of his mouth, in between gasps for air, with his left hand raised as if he was waiting to be called upon, he told me that for two and one half years, between 1996 and 1998, he stayed in bed 24 h a day, 7 days a week except on Saturdays when he would meet her. He loved going out to local restaurants with his mother and when she would take him shopping to provide him with necessities which were meant to hold him over until she would see him again. Before her death 12 years ago from cancer, she had found him an apartment where he would live for the next 5 years. When his mother died, he became the recipient of a small trust fund that she set up to help him. This, along with his monthly social security income and medical assistance, makes it a little easier for him to get by, but he wouldn't agree that he lives comfortably.

For a while Ted seemed to be succeeding. He volunteered doing clerical work for the Alliance for the Mentally Ill, completed a case management-training program and attended a transitional psychiatric day program. In addition, he enjoys visiting his brother and sister who live many states away. "It's an excuse to do something different, different from my everyday routine." But the TD raged on. He would soon stop driving, while continuing to volunteer his services wherever he could.

He longs for contact with people. With an apathetic face and tremulous right hand secondary to the parkinsonian side effects of antipsychotic medications, he told me of having no wife, girlfriend, or children. I was reminded of this one day when I met Ted while getting a cup of coffee at a shop a few blocks from my office. In the corner of the store, sitting by himself, I saw him resting, eyes closed in a big overstuffed crushed velvet chair with his hand relaxed around a paper cup on the table next to him. I had never seen him so peaceful. Perhaps he is only at peace when asleep I wondered. I debated whether or not to disturb him but decided to touch his forearm lightly. He lurched as he opened his eyes and we chatted for a few minutes. As I went to leave he said "Hey Doc. Thanks for stopping by and saying hello."

As if his mental and physical problems weren't enough, Ted, like many who live in an inner city also suffers from the stress that comes from fear for his own safety. His apartment has been vandalized five times over a course of 4 years. He has been verbally threatened with physical harm and is repeatedly taunted by groups of teenagers who laugh at the difficulties he has with talking or breathing. He has been pelted with rocks and stones as he walked on his sidewalk, been shot in the face with a bb gun while using a pay phone and robbed at gunpoint six times over a course of 13 years.

The Austrian psychiatrist Viktor Emil Frankl (1905–1997) was held prisoner during World War II at the Theresienstadt concentration camp. He wondered why some living under such terrible physical and emotional conditions survived and others seemed to quickly succumb to their torture. In his book *Man's Search for Meaning* he offers an explanation [4]. Frankl writes those who survived shared a commonality of having found meaning in their life. Those who survived were living for someone, for some cause, or had come to understand the meaning behind their suffering. I thought of Ted and how he also has suffered terribly, yet has seemingly found meaning in his life.

When I asked him what his sources of hope were, he almost seemed surprised by the question and hesitated before saying, "I don't want to die. I take each day as it comes." He went to explain, "I am not religious. I don't believe in Jesus or a higher power. Although raised Jewish I don't identify or affiliate. I believe in a better world. A world that can get better. I've seen it's gotten better—a little better." Despite having many reasons to be negative, he had a positive outlook on life. He told me his sources of pleasure now are food, looking at good-looking women, visits with his brother and sister, and volunteer work. He believes in supporting patients' rights and has volunteered to serve on the committee of a local psychiatric hospital, along with most any patient care related volunteer job he could find. When I asked him why he volunteers, particularly helping others with mental illness he cited, "Because I am good at it. Very good at it. I am organized, meticulous, (and) effective." From all the jobs I've done I get good references... driving, clerical, going to nursing homes, helping the indigent and the poor."

In researching TD further I learned that it is often mild and reversible. The number of those who develop severe and irreversible TD is low considering the number of those on long-term antipsychotic therapy. Furthermore, this problem has been reduced even further with the discovery and broad use of atypical antipsychotics. There is controversy as to whether the incidence has really gone down. I was told by a colleague in neurology at my institution that some new medications have shown some promise in helping those with TD.

Ted was elated to be offered a same day appointment when I called to see if I could get him in to see this motor disorders specialist. After his evaluation I learned that Ted suffered from a curious movement disorder which might be made better by one of several anticholinergic medications. The concern we both had was would he take them. Ted was given a prescription for Trihexyphenidyl.

It's been 1 month since Ted was prescribed a new psychiatric medication. He told me by phone today that he hasn't started it yet. "I am reluctant to take it. I don't think it will cure tardive dyskinesia. What do you think?" he asked. I told Ted we could talk about it when he comes in tomorrow for his blood pressure check. I knew that given all the suffering he had been through, including the adverse effects of medications meant to help him, that I could not convince him or myself that this new one would clearly be different.

Viktor Frankl would tell us that Ted will be OK because he has found meaning in his life. "Those who have a 'why' to live, can bear with almost any 'how'."

References

1. Osler W. The student life. Aequanimitas: with other addresses to medical students, nurses and practitioners of medicine. Philadelphia, PA: P. Blackiston's Son and Co.; 1907. p. 404–5.
2. Wagner-Martin L. William Carlos Williams: a reference guide. USA: G K Hall & Co; 1978.
3. Reeve C. The Christopher Reeve Homepage, "We, the people". <http://www.chrisreevehomepage.com/editorial-wethepeople.html>. Accessed May 2009.
4. Frankl VE. Man's search for meaning. An introduction to logotherapy. Boston: Beacon, Random House; 1946.

Searching for the True Poetry of Life

Colgan R. I am sorry I was late. Acad Med. 2002;77(10):946.
Williams W. The doctor stories. New York: New Directions Publishing Corporation; 1984.

A Meaningful Life

Tarsy D, Lungu C, Baldessarini RJ. Epidemiology of tardive dyskinesia before and during the era of modern antipsychotic drugs. Handb Clin Neurol. 2011;100:601–16.
Tarsy D, Baldessarini RJ. Epidemiology of tardive dyskinesia: is risk declining with modern antipsychotics? Mov Disord. 2006;21(5):589–98. Review.
Frankl VE. Man's search for meaning. An introduction to logotherapy. Boston: Beacon, Random House

A Doctor's Journal

Taylor RB. Medical writing: a guide for clinicians, educators, and researchers. New York: Springer; 2011.

University of Iowa Carver College of Medicine. Examined life: writing and the art of medicine. Writers Workshop, held in April each year. www.medicine.uiowa.edu/md/writing

Chapter 10
Heal Thyself

I have known doctors (including a gastroenterologist) who were diagnosed with advanced colon cancers due to lack of proper colorectal cancer screening. I know physicians who care for adult patients but do not know their own blood pressure or cholesterol level. When you care for yourself or loved ones, it becomes difficult to draw the line and even easier to overstep those drawn by professional medical societies and ethics committees. When you or a loved one is sick, seek out another physician for treatment.

One summer, I served as an "able-bodied" seaman for the Association of Maryland Pilots. One night near Norfolk, Virginia, I assisted a Chesapeake Bay pilot to the ship's ladder at 2 a.m., amidst gale-force winds raging up the bay. As the 30-ft launch heaved up and down alongside this inbound container ship, I had difficulty tying the bag to the rope needed to carry it topside. We both were in danger of going overboard. The senior pilot urged me to look out for myself while performing the dangerous tasks required by this job. He yelled to me through the wind, "One hand for yourself and one hand for the ship."

This maritime adage applies to us in medicine as well. Healers should not feel guilty about looking after themselves, even if doing so comes before delivery of care to their patients. By being healthy ourselves, we may live another day to take good care of our patients and make sure the care we provide is the most effective and successful possible. My advice is that healers should find someone they have confidence in and seek their care. Be it preventive or treatment, you have the right to receive expert care. Your patients deserve to have you at the peak of wellness, so that you can best serve them. Too often, physicians—being in conveniently close proximity to medical

R. Colgan, *Advice to the Healer: On the Art of Caring*,
DOI 10.1007/978-1-4614-5170-9_10,
© Springer Science+Business Media, LLC 2013

care—will self-diagnose and treat themselves. Even worse, they extend this care to their family. Although most of us do this to some extent, it starts us down the path to crossing those lines. In treating our loved ones, we are unable to be objective and less likely to be as thorough. The care we provide to them is skewed by our connection, and often it is substandard to care provided by someone else. The best way a physician can heal himself is to seek the advice of a trusted healer and follow it.

Another important way to look after yourself is to realize that in any service industry, including health care, you may find yourself in threatening situations. Fortunately this is rare in most fields of medicine, but as a public servant we may sometimes be confronted with people who look to harm us. Two true stories from my career help to illustrate this point. Some patients are overly friendly because that is their nature or the way they express appreciation. Other patients are overly friendly because of mental illness. I admire the intent of physicians who give out their home and cell phone numbers or provide their home addresses so that patients may easily contact them. I admit to doing this rarely because I have seen firsthand how mental illness can distort a patient's interpretation of reality and social boundaries. I was stalked by one of my patients, and I wouldn't wish this experience on anyone. What follows is an account of this interaction, which I am anxious to tell you about for one reason only: I hope you never have to go through what I went through.

For privacy reasons, I will go out of my way to not be specific in the details of this interaction. Suffice it to say that I saw a patient in my private practice years ago for a rather straightforward complaint and recommended an appropriate, standard of care evaluation and management plan. This was followed by several back and forth interactions with this patient that grew increasingly bizarre. I became concerned. I couldn't understand why I was receiving single-spaced, multiple-paged letters by this patient alleging mistreatment and malpractice. I was threatened with being reported to several oversight agencies for my bad doctoring. I felt then, as I know now, that I had done nothing wrong. I had the foresight to discharge the patient from my practice in proper legal format, i.e., in writing, with 30 days' notice and offering to forward medical records to another physician upon receipt of a written directive to do so. Nonetheless, the patient continued to stalk me by phone, mail, and in person, informing me that the discharge was not accepted until I righted the perceived wrong that I had done. I began to fear for my family's safety, as I thought this person was truly out of his mind.

The nightmare didn't end with personal intimidation, however. I was reported to the State Board of Physicians, a federal office that dealt with the rights of those with disabilities, and my state's medical assistance office. I sought the counsel of an attorney. Once I told him my story, he reached into his bookshelf and pulled down a state law text. The attorney opened to a page describing in detail what was happening to me; it was the state law on harassment.

I was advised that I could go before a judge and get a restraining order. I reflected upon what I had learned in behavioral pediatrics, as I thought this person's behaviors were childlike and at a minimum represented a type of acting out. I did not know then with certainty that the person was certifiably mentally ill. I remembered that if you want to extinguish a certain behavior in a child, it is better to not attend to the behavior but rather to ignore it. I decided against pursuing the restraining order, as I thought it might add fuel to the fire. Two months later this patient was admitted for his first paranoid schizophrenic break, which was later followed by many more psychiatric hospitalizations. In retrospect, my patient's abnormal pursuit of me represented the early signs of psychiatric illness. This taught me an important lesson: Physician—protect yourself.

Protecting yourself is not self-centered but represents good medical practice. The example above is, of course, extreme, but there are many ways to avoid or abate dangerous situations should they arise. Examples include sitting near an open door when you perceive a patient to be hostile or making sure to have an attendant present—of the opposite sex—when performing sensitive parts of the physical exam (e.g., the pelvic or genital exam). Additionally, you want to be careful when examining an acutely psychotic paranoid schizophrenic patient. Be careful not to be perceived as threatening, and, if need be, simply stop the exam and walk away. I declined to examine a patient like this when requested to perform the admission exam at a local psychiatric hospital, diffusing the situation to avoid the possibility of physician harm. Instead I spoke with him in the hallway, where I could exit easily. During the exam, I was struck by how paranoid he appeared. After asking him if I may listen to his back, I noticed his spine straightened, and he became very rigid. Something told me that I should be frightened of this unfortunate patient. I concluded the exam and thanked him for his time. The next day, I was asked to attend to the same psychiatric hospital's staff psychiatrist, who suffered a stab to the neck from the very same patient. She had come physically too close to this patient and was unable to protect herself when he snapped. I believe there is no greater satisfaction than to serve, but the wise healer recognizes that he or she must be in good physical condition in order to serve well and is aware that there will be rare instances when you must be mindful of your own personal safety.

Reference

1. Woodward T. Make room for sentiment. Baltimore, MD: University of Maryland Medical Alumni Association; 1998.

Further Reading and Resource

Angres D. et al. Healing the healer: the addicted physician. Madison, CT: Psychosocial Press; 2001.

Chapter 11
The Healer

Je le pansais, Dieu le guérit.
I bandaged them, God healed them.

—Ambroise Paré [1]

What does the consummate, flawless healer look like? We do not and cannot know, because he or she does not exist. Just as we cannot define what perfection or pure beauty is, we must reconcile that any declaration of such is not a fact, but an opinion. Throughout the ages, many great teachers of the art of caring have both spoken about and lived exemplary lives that demonstrate what most of us—from both the clinical and lay communities—would likely agree is the essence of the consummate healer. While it may be difficult to define the art of caring, most people can often tell you that they know it when they see it. But where is this notion written?

The clinician who strives to make the transition from technician to healer deserves to be educated as to what makes a great healer. He or she must take this journey to improve his or her own abilities and, if for no other reason, to know what gold standard to aspire to. Even if perfection is not obtainable in the pursuit of the ideal clinician–patient relationship, we owe it to our patients to attempt to define this concept as it embodies the art of caring. Moreover, once this bar is made visible, we have a duty to try to achieve this level of care even if we fail. We must strive for perfection for the betterment of our patients.

The young healer might reasonably ask, "Who do I turn to for advice?" I suggest that we begin by identifying role models known to each of us, whether we are a student, young physician, or more seasoned clinician. These are the "ordinary" physicians in our community who on a daily basis are doing the extraordinary by practicing

R. Colgan, *Advice to the Healer: On the Art of Caring*,
DOI 10.1007/978-1-4614-5170-9_11,
© Springer Science+Business Media, LLC 2013

medicine in an exceptional manner with little fame. In addition to the wisdom of our peers, we should also take in the wisdom, teachings, and examples of those who have been recognized as distinguished and honored leaders. No one person can accurately scan the history of clinical care and create a list of "best practices" on which all clinicians would agree.

Despite this, I do not think we should abandon such a quest, as quixotic as it may sound. Then again, maybe like Don Quixote, I am delusional. Perhaps Osler had this in mind when he urged medical students to read Cervantes' *Don Quixote*. The hero of this epic novel acted upon erroneous fixed beliefs that seemed unreal and unachievable to those around him, while proclaiming proudly:

> It is the mission of each true knight…
> His duty… nay, his privilege!
> To dream the impossible dream,
> To fight the unbeatable foe,
> To bear with unbearable sorrow
> To run where the brave dare not go;
> To right the unrightable wrong [2].

To anyone who believes that the absolutes of patient care are not captured in such poetic advice: I wholeheartedly agree with you. I urge others to improve how we teach today's young clinicians to be superb healers and, moreover, that these lessons are made applicable to common situations encountered in practice. This is not to say I do not appreciate the connection between these poetic teachings and modern clinical practice. However, I offer this book as one physician's effort to carry forth this important and humanistic dialogue which began centuries ago. We may come to better understand how to practice the art of caring by looking to the thoughts, writings, and histories of Imhotep, Hippocrates, Aristotle, and Plato in the Ancient era; The Three Divine Doctors of Jian An, Rhazes, Avicenna, and Maimonides in Medieval times; Nightingale, Osler, Schweitzer, Peabody, and Rogers in the twentieth century; and some of today's modern masters including Pellegrino, Farmer, and Woodward.

But before we can effectively teach the art of caring we must identify what it is. In medicine, physicians are not the sole interpreters of what constitutes the ideal physician–patient relationship. Those in the nonmedical community have and should always weigh in on what they value in their doctor, for it is those patients we largely serve. Once we better understand what values and behaviors are cherished by our patients, we can teach these lessons to the young technician who strives to be a true healer.

> …To love, pure and chaste, from afar,
> To try, when your arms are too weary,
> To reach the unreachable star! [2]

Throughout time and to the present day, cultures value the good health of their people. As healers, we are in a fortunate position to improve the health and well-being of those we care for. Because of this, we are treated differently—in fact better—and we are rewarded for our hard work and recognized for attempting to better humankind. These rewards come in both tangible and intangible forms. Most healers need never be concerned about a mortgage or a car payment. We can typically go out to dinner without worrying about the cost. But, as noted in the Bible in the book of Luke, "Much will be required from everyone to whom much has been given. But even more will be demanded from the one to whom much has been entrusted" [3].

True healers understand that medicine is not just a job but a call to service, a vocation. It has been said that some doctors suffer from a "God complex," arrogantly thinking themselves above or better than their patients. The role of the physician naturally sets up a disparity in power and knowledge between those giving and receiving care. Unfortunately this power is sometimes abused. We must strive to be humble and grateful for our position in society. Hippocrates sets this record straight, noting in *Decorum*, "The gods are the real physicians" [4]. Likewise we are reminded by the French surgeon Ambroise Paré (1510–1590) that our abilities as physicians are limited—that God heals and we supply the bandages [1]. However, it is not as simple as this. We must still learn how to apply the bandages, to practice the science and art of caring with a goal of perfection, in recognition of our privilege.

In researching the lives and behaviors of some of history's greatest healers, I noticed that several themes recur throughout the eras. These luminaries are in agreement on several characteristics of the ideal healer, which can be clearly defined through their writings or exemplified by their convictions and the principles by which they lived. The essential attributes of the healer can be viewed in terms of (1) the healer as a person; (2) the healer–patient interaction; and (3) healing as a vocation. Below, I've pulled together some thoughts on what constitutes the ideal clinician in each of these areas.

...This is my Quest to follow that star,
No matter how hopeless, no matter how far,
To fight for the right
Without question or pause,
To be willing to march into hell
For a heavenly cause! [2]

The Healer as a Person

A healer is a moral agent who cares for others based upon altruistic conviction. He/she is one who shows respect not only to patients but to family, acquaintances, and self. A healer is described by others as someone who is above all civil, polite, and kind in all interactions, regardless of a person's station in life. He or she is able to detach from the allure of worldly pleasures so as to be the best healer possible, while remaining humble and knowing the limitations of this exceptional art.

I recently asked a group of medical students to describe a healer's personal attributes. They described him or her as someone who was empathetic, selfless, giving, and personable. This healer was depicted as hard working, a constant learner who is respectful, approachable, thoughtful, compassionate, honest, and caring. Other noted qualities included kindness, being nonjudgmental, wisdom, being realistic as well as idealistic, understanding, patience, curiosity, and an ability to maintain a broad perspective and an open mind.

...And I know, if I'll only be true
To this glorious Quest,
That my heart will lie peaceful and calm
When I'm laid to my rest [2].

The Healer–Patient Interaction

A healer can be seen by others as someone who cares for patients and focuses on them, particularly when no one is watching. This person understands that if it is not possible to help someone, then at a minimum we should "first do no harm." The healer goes out of his or her way to learn from all patients and others who aid in their care. He or she is observant, thorough, methodical, contemplative, and careful.

The healer is an independent thinker who practices evidence-based medicine, nursing, dentistry, social work, psychology, or another clinical field. The healer does so in the context of providing the most appropriate and effective care possible.

Under stressful situations, the healer exhibits both an inner and outer calmness in the discharge of duties. Healers are not easily flustered or perturbed. All matters between clinician and patient are kept confidential and the patient's trust is preserved at all times. The healer looks to educate patients on how to improve their health while remaining open enough to learn from them. The consummate healer recognizes that he or she is caring for someone with a disease, and this illness affects both the patient and possibly the patient's family as well. The healer is temperate and modest in making recommendations. When it comes to therapeutics, he or she is assistive to nature and when felt to be beneficial, looks to incorporate proper diet, exercise, and the patient's activities in the overall care of the patient. Above all else, the healer strives for excellence in every physician–patient relationship.

When I asked the same group of medical students to describe what they would expect to see in the interactions between a healer and his or her patient, they imagined a healer that is skilled in listening to patients and who avoids interruption. This ideal healer is empathetic, is respectful, maintains excellent rapport, and demonstrates a good and wholesome sense of humor. Other attributes they expect of this healing relationship are displayed as the physician ensures patient comfort and allows for two-way communication that establishes a sense of equality between the physician and patient. Moreover, this relationship is used in an effective way to not only address the patient's health concerns, but to assure that his or her emotional needs are also being addressed. This ideal healer helps channel a patient's fears and frustrations into hope and action, and accomplishes this while being honest, trustful, and showing a genuine interest in the patient as a person.

The Healer's Vocation

Someone who has made the transition from technician to healer looks beyond his or her own needs. This individual recognizes that there is more to caring than the finite number of individual patients seen throughout his or her lifetime. While each patient is of utmost importance, an exemplary healer is one who also views the betterment of humankind as a personal responsibility. Where inequality in health care exists, the healer accepts the challenge to do what is possible to help society as a whole, particularly those who represent the most vulnerable and disadvantaged populations. The healer acknowledges a personal accountability for his or her actions, not only to the patients that he or she directly serves but also to the entire community. The healer provides care for the poor and advocates for those who are victimized by healthcare disparities. This is accomplished by diligent observation of patterns of disease amongst the patient population. The ideal healer aims to educate current and future healers. Furthermore, the ideal healer inspires enduring leadership, volunteers in his or her community, and is a pacifist and an environmentalist. He or she works past social prejudices and provides equal care to all patients, regardless of race, ethnicity, or social background. This person demonstrates love for others by a commitment to service. As an ideal healer, he or she shows respect and honor to the teachers and mentors in the practice of the art and science of medicine.

Simply put, the art of caring is showing love to your fellow man through your unique skillset. I've written much about the details of how to practice this art, but in the end it really is quite simple. So simple, in fact, that a 12-year-old boy could fully grasp it.

Nkosi Johnson (1989–2001) was born HIV-positive in a township of Johannesburg. He has been called one of South Africa's "Greats" by putting a face to the multitude of people around the world who suffer with the AIDS virus. At the age of two, he was adopted by Gail Johnson, a Johannesburg Public Relations professional, when his mother was no longer able to care for him. His biological mother soon thereafter died of AIDS.

Nkosi came to public attention after being denied admission to a primary school because of his HIV-positive status. He later won the hearts of millions around the world when, as a keynote speaker to the 13th International AIDS Conference, he encouraged acceptance by those who were HIV-negative to remember that they are not so different:

> Care for us and accept us—we are all human beings. We are normal. We have hands. We have feet. We can walk, we can talk, we have needs just like everyone else—don't be afraid of us—we are all the same! [5]

Nkosi's life story was profiled in Jim Wooten's book *We Are All the Same*. At the end of one of the interviews, Nkosi reminded the reporter that he had not asked about the boy's impending death. What Nkosi said next might be good advice for everyone to follow, but seems particularly appropriate for those who are looking to serve:

> Do all you can with what you have in the time you have in the place you are [6].

I encourage all clinicians to embrace the science of their respective discipline and to stay current with the evolving evidence-based practice of their field of expertise. If we never forget to focus on the quality of care we render to each of our patients, we will likely practice the art of caring to the best of our abilities. Above all else, be cognizant that your vocation is a sacred and honorable one. We are privileged to watch over our fellow man, to use the lessons bestowed by those who came before us to provide every member of our human family with thoughtful and compassionate medical care.

> …and the world will be better for this,
> That one man, scorned and covered with scars,
> Still strove, with his last ounce of courage,
> To reach the unreachable stars! [2]

The Doctor—Sir Luke Fildes

Victorian artist Sir Luke Fildes' (1843–1927) painting *The Doctor* (1887, The Tate Britain, London) leads the viewer to understand without words what a caring doctor is and how he was viewed by the painter in this pre-antibiotic era of medicine. (See Fig. 11.1)

The painting depicts the ideals of medicine. The viewer is immediately drawn to the image of a well-to-do physician who has made a house call to the cottage of a laborer to care for his sick child. Perhaps most striking is the intensity of the gaze of the doctor as he patiently sits and attends. The child's eyes are closed as she lays on a makeshift bed of two nonmatching chairs, her left hand neither fully opened nor closed as if to signify she is hanging on for dear life. We don't know if she is about to die or if she has turned the corner toward getting better. Next to the doctor's table are a pestle and mortar, a cup, and many crumpled pieces of paper which suggest there have been multiple efforts to get her curative medicinal potion right. The child's

Fig. 11.1 Sir Luke Fildes' painting, *The Doctor*, © Tate London, 2012; used with permission

mother can be seen in the corner of the room with her head down, perhaps sobbing. The father is looking off into the distance with one arm rested on his wife's shoulder in an effort to console her. But there is hope. The glimmer of morning light filtering in through the window hints that a new dawn has arrived and, with it, the potential for betterment. Fildes' first son died of tuberculosis on Christmas morning in 1877. One theory behind *The Doctor* is that it represents the lasting impression Fildes' family doctor made on the artist as he took care of his dying son.

R.S. Downie includes a picture of *The Doctor* in his illustrated anthology *The Healing Arts*. Downie comments: "This painting is an eloquent portrayal of what medicine is all about—the doctor, the patient, and the quality of the relationship that exists between them. The physician is attending the patient, watching and waiting—being there. Much of the painting's impact is the space between the physician's eyes and the child, which is filled, solely, by the patient's gaze" [7]. Jane Moore in the *British Journal of General Practice* rightfully adds: "Most importantly, Fildes' timeless painting, *The Doctor*, reminds contemporary doctors of the crucial importance of the relationship between a patient and the doctor and the value of a patient-centered approach" [8].

A Healer's Prayer

Though these thoughts on healing have been organized into a prayer, they could just as easily be adapted into a quiet meditation on your career or a set of principles to guide you through your day.

> Let me begin each clinical encounter by always putting my patient's needs first. Grant me the strength to not be seduced by the allure of worldly pleasures, so as to be the best healer I can be, as I look to be thorough and careful in practicing my art.

> Guide me as I practice this sacred vocation. May I have the wisdom to learn from the lessons of my teachers as I contemplate how to best serve each person who seeks my counsel. Help me to use all of my senses as I strive for excellence in caring for my patients and to understand that if I cannot help someone, then at a minimum I will do no harm. Strengthen me to have an inner and outer calmness when faced with the inevitable difficulties that lie before me.

> Show me how to best educate my patients on how to live longer and healthier lives, while being open to learning from those whom I serve. Show me how to be temperate and modest as I look to assist nature by incorporating proper diet, exercise and my patient's own resources in his or her overall care. Never let me forget that I am caring for someone who is suffering from a disease and not taking care of a disease. May I never forget my duty to care based upon a conviction of pursuing altruistic beneficence, marked by showing compassion for others as I commit myself to a life of service.

> May I not abandon, but look to serve the poor and advocate for those who suffer because of disparities in our health care system. Remind me to keep matters between my patient and myself confidential and that I am accountable for my actions. May I always show respect and care for myself and my family, while being kind in my everyday interactions with others.

> I ask for humility in knowing the limitations of my art. May I always end each encounter with my patient knowing that I have done my best in assisting the patient by applying the bandages, while taking comfort in the fact that only power greater than me heals.

References

1. Keynes G. The apologie and treatise of Ambroise Paré containing the voyages made into divers, with many of his writings upon surgery. Chicago, IL: University of Chicago Press; 1952.
2. De Cervantes M. Don Quijote. Ed. (Trans: de Armas Wilson D). Burton Raffel. Norton critical. 2nd ed. New York: W.W. Norton and Co.; 1999.
3. Luke. http://bible.cc/luke/12-48.htm. Accessed 9 Sep 2009.
4. Adams F, The genuine works of Hippocrates. Baltimore, Williams & Wilkins Co.; 1939.
5. http://en.wikiquote.org/wiki/Nkosi_Johnson. Accessed 2 May 2012.
6. Wooten J. We are all the same. 1st ed. New York: Penguin Press HC; 2004.
7. Downie RS. The healing arts. Oxford: Oxford University Press; 1994.
8. Moore J. What the 1887 painting The Doctor can teach us about the practice of medicine today. Br J Gen Pract. 2008;58(548):210–3.

Further Reading and Resources

Sulmasy D. The healers calling: a spirituality for physicians and other health care professionals. Mahwah, NJ: Paulist Press; 1997.

The Institute for the Study of Health and Illness. <http://www.commonweal.org/ishi/>

Downie RS. The healing arts. Oxford: Oxford University Press; 1994.

Moore J. What the 1887 painting The Doctor can teach us about the practice of medicine today. Br J Gen Pract. 2008;58(548):210–3.

Wooten J. We are all the same. 1st ed. New York: Penguin Press HC; 2004.

Index

A
Adams, Francis, 13
American Medical Association
        (AMA), 87
Aphorisms, 15
Arbuthnot, John, 1
Art of caring, 2
Art of presentation, younger clinicians
        assessments, 108
        cardiologist, 103
        care providers, 104
        common mistakes, 108–109
        components, shortness of breath, 108
        HPI, 105–106
        language of medicine, 105
        for medicine, 103
        nursing, 103
        objective exam, 106
        obstetrician, 104
        Osler's admonition, 104
        primary care medicine, 107
        risk factors, CAD, 103–104
Avicenna (Ibn Sina), 35–37

B
BATHE technique
        bad situations, 130
        love and acceptance, 131
        15-min therapeutic hour, 130–131
        therapeutic skills adoption
                paradigm, 130
Biers, Bob, 10

Browning, Robert, 7
Bryan, Charles S., 58, 63–65

C
CAD. *See* Coronary artery disease
        (CAD)
Chinese and medieval medicine
        Avicenna (Ibn Sina), 35–37
        Feng, Dong, 31–32
        Maimonides, Moses, 37–42
        Rhazes (Abu Bakr Muhammad ibn
                Zakariya Razi), 32–35
        Tuo, Hua, 30–31
        Zhongjing, Zhang, 29–30
Civility
        effective health care delivery, 117
        etiquette-based medicine, 118–119
        habits, physicians, 118
        interactions with patients, 117
        physician behavior, patient
                attitudes, 118
        rules (*see* Rules, healers)
Clinician as counselor
        description, 127
        freedom, pressure/coercion, 129
        teaching tools, 15-min therapy, 129
        therapeutic relationship,
                permissiveness, 128
        time, 129
        unconditional positive regards,
                127–128
        "win-win" situation, 128

R. Colgan, *Advice to the Healer: On the Art of Caring*,
DOI 10.1007/978-1-4614-5170-9,
© Springer Science+Business Media, LLC 2013

Colgan, Richard, 146
Coronary artery disease (CAD),
      103–104
Corpus Hippocraticum, 13
Cushing, Harvey, 60, 62

D
de Cervantes, Miquel, 23, 162
Doctor's Journal
      apologizing, 143–146
      meaningful life, 150–154
      modern family, 147–150
      poems, private practice, 142
      recollections, 140–142
      true poetry of life, 139–140
Dossey, Barbara, 46, 49
Downie, R.S., 168

E
Early Greeks, 22–25
Enoch Pratt Library, 148
Evidence-based medicine, 3

F
Farmer, Paul
      clinician-patient relationship, 91
      commercialization, health care,
            92–93
      "conventional medicine", 94
      healer's duty, 94
      Mountains Beyond Mountains, 90
      Pathologies of Power, 92
      physician, medical-anthropologist
            and health advocate, 89–90
      societal shortcomings, 93–94
      structural violence, 93
      TB epidemics, 92
Feng, Dong, 31–32
Fildes, Luke, 167–169
Filomena, Santa, 50–51
Florence Nightingale
      born, 45
      cared, people, 45–46
      care, wounded and sick, 46
      contributions, 48

Coxcomb diagram, 47–48
      "health of houses", 47
      "lady with lamp", 46
      list of accomplishments, 46
      notes on nursing, art of caring,
            48–50
      "pesthouses" and improved
            sanitation, 47
      physicians, dentists and
            pharmacists, 48
Forni, P., 118, 119, 124
Frankl, Viktor Emil, 153, 154

G
Gallagher, T., 121
Good communication, younger
            clinicians, 112–113

H
Hammurabi
      art of medicine, 12
      healers, 12
      history, 11–12
      physician–patient interaction, 12
Hartshorne, Henry, 4
Healer–patient interaction, 164–165
Healers
      attributes, 163–164
      description, 161
      disparity, power and knowledge,
            163
      Fildes, Luke, 167–169
      healer–patient interaction,
            164–165
      lessons, young technician, 163
      objectives, 161–162
      as person, 164
      physician–patient relationship, 162
      poetic advice, 162
      prayer, 169
      vocation (*see* Healer's vocation)
Healer's prayer, 169
Healer's vocation
      art and science of medicine, 166
      evidence-based practice, 167
      HIV-positive status, 166–167

personal responsibility, 165–166
thoughtful and compassionate
    medical care, 167
Healing professions, 2, 3
Health Insurance Privacy and
    Portability Act (HIPPA), 19
Heal thyself
    "able-bodied" seaman, 157
    advanced colon cancers, 157
    behavioral pediatrics, 159
    care of physicians, 158
    delivery of care, patients, 157
    good medical practice, 159
    peak of wellness, 157
    personal intimidation, 159
    for private practice, 158
    psychiatric hospital's staff
        psychiatrist, 159–160
    in threatening situations, 158
HIPPA. See Health Insurance
    Privacy and Portability
    Act (HIPPA)
Hippocrates
    Aphorisms, 15
    attitudes and expectations,
        patient's, 15–16
    Corpus Hippocraticum, 13
    Hippocratic Oath (see Hippocratic
        Oath)
    honest on human frailties, 16
    medicine's application essay, 17
    non-physicians, 17
    power of observation, 14
    "professionals", 17
    quotes, 13
    scientific validation, 14–15
    society experience health care
        disparities, 16
Hippocratic Oath
    art of diagnosis, 20–21
    facial look of dying, 21–22
    health and health care
        expectations, 18
    HIPPA, 19
    malpractice, 21
    passion, 19
    patient and health care
        providers, 19

physician–patient confidentiality,
    19
prognostic indications, poor
    patient outcome, 21
teachings, centuries of
    scrutiny, 22
History of present illness (HPI)
    description, 104
    medical history, medications and
        allergies, 106
    newspaper article, 105
    shortness of breath/dyspnea, 105
HPI. See History of present illness
    (HPI)
Humanistic patient-centered
    care, 2

I
Imhotep (2655–2600 BC)
    broken bones and perils, crocodile
        bites, 10
    historical figure, 9
    magical thinking, 9–10
    philosopher, 9
    physicians, 11
    scientific practices, 11
    Surgical Papyrus, 10
Ioannidis, J.P.A., 90, 91

J
Jian An
    description, 29
    Feng, Dong, 31–32
    Tuo, Hua, 30–31
    Zhongjing, Zhang, 29–30

K
Kahn, Michael W., 117, 118, 124
Kalamazoo consensus statement,
    113–114
Kidder, Tracy, 90, 91

L
Lieberman, Joseph A., 129, 131

M

Mackowiak, Phillip, 49

Maimonides, Moses
  Arabic medicine, 37, 38
  devotion, patients and passion, 38
  physician–patient relationship, 39
  physician's oath and prayer, 39–41
  theologian, 38

Makoul, Gregory, 114

Malpractice, 131–132

Medical educators, 5

Medical ethics
  caring, 88
  "focus on the patient", 88–89
  humanistic characteristics, 89
  physician, 87–88
  role model of physician, 89
  true leader, 88
  unified notion of care, 89

Meyer, Marvin, 72

Missed acute abdomen, 133

Missed myocardial ischemia, 132–133

Modern family
  case description, 147
  Enoch Pratt Library, 148
  facial twitches and motor
      disturbances, 146–147
  humility, perseverance and grace,
      149
  Joe, inner-city hospital, 146
  nontraditional family, 149
  psychiatric institutionalization, 148
  spider-like microscope, 149
  workup, chest pain, 148–149

Modern Masters
  access, 99
  care for the patient, 99–100
  elasticity, 98–99
  Gift of Time, 97–98
  Paul Farmer (*see* Farmer, Paul)
  Pellegrino, Edmund D (*see*
      Pellegrino, Edmund D.)
  principles, medical ethics (*see*
      Medical ethics)
  unsung heroes and heroines
      description, 94–95
      primacy, trusted healing
          relationship, 95–97

Woodward, Theodore E (*see*
    Woodward, Theodore E.)

Moore, Jane, 168

Mosby, C.V., 49

O

Oath of Maimonides, 39–40

Osler, Sir William
  aequanimaty, 53
  "art of detachment", 55
  auscultation, 56, 58
  cardinal concepts, 52
  care carefully
      description, 63–64
      "do the kind thing and do it
          first", 64
      power of observation, 65
      qualities/excellence taught and
          modeled, 65
      simplicity and temperance, 64
      state-of-the-art care, 64
  clinical rotation, 53–54
  contemplation, 56, 60
  English-speaking physician, 51
  ER attending physician
      question, 54
  father of internal medicine, 51
  "grace of humility", 56
  imperturbability, 52–53
  inspection, 56, 57
  inspiration, great physician, 58
  Institute of Medicine, 56
  learn and teach, 63
  manipulation of a catheter, 54
  mentors, 61–62
  occurrence and reoccurrence,
      57–58
  palpation, 56, 59
  physiology and disease
      process, 52
  "prince of friends and
      benefactors", 62–63
  teacher and student, 55
  time management, 59–61
  true to certain ideals, 61
  types of lymphoma, 54–55
  "virtue of method", 55

P

Peabody, Francis Weld
  American medical educator, 66
  atypical migraine-like
      headaches, 68
  care of the patient, 66–67
  functional disorders, 68
  functional illnesses and
      psychosomatic disorders, 68
  functional/psychosomatic
      disorder, 67
  inpatient medicine description, 67
Pellegrino, Edmund D.
  AMA, 87
  bioethics and philosophy of
      medicine, 81
  business community, medicine, 83
  cardinal virtues, 84
  The Commodification of Medical
      and Health Care, 82–83
  "consumers" and "providers", 83
  contemporary medicine, 87
  dubious procedures, tests/
      supplements, 84
  ethical path, physicians, 83–84
  journal of medicine and
      philosophy, 81
  moral agent, 84
  "non-philosopher philosopher", 82
  *A Philosophical Reconstruction of
      Medical Morality and the
      Caring Ethic*, 86
  physician-educators, 80–81
  physician-patient relationship,
      81–82, 86
  "the art of medicine", 81
  true paternalistic manner, 86–87
  virtuous healer, 85
  virtuous physician, 85
Physician–patient relationship, 3, 5
Plato, 82, 84
Poems, private practice, 142
Porter, Roy, 13, 20
Prayer of Maimonides, 40–42
Private practice
  academic exercise, 136
  clinician as counselor (*see*
      Clinician as counselor)
  common lawsuits, 132
  defense *vs.* malpractice allegations,
      135
  failure, informing patients,
      133–134
  good practice, 131
  "how to BATHE your patients as
      you SOAP them" (*see*
      BATHE technique)
  insurance carrier and attorney's
      office, 136
  litigation process, 136
  malpractice, 131–132
  malpractice defendants, 134
  medical errors, 136
  missed acute abdomen, 133
  "missed" diagnosis/"bad
      outcome", 134
  missed myocardial ischemia,
      132–133
  patient's medical record, 135
  preliminary legal challenge,
      134–135

R

Ramon y Cajal, Santiago, 3
Recollections, poetic moments
  Gregory B., 140–141
  Margaret R., 141–142
  Stephanie B., 141
Reeve, Christopher, 145
Rhazes (Abu Bakr Muhammad ibn
      Zakariya Razi)
  daily routines, doctors, 34
  disciplines, 33
  evidence-based medicine,
      middle ages, 34
  fever and urinary ailments, 34
  importance, sound mind
      and body, 35
  influential alchemist, 32–33
  meticulous observation and
      constant questioning, 33
  power of observation, 33
  professional medical care, 35
Rodin, A., 7
Rogers, Carl R., 127–129, 131

Rules, healers
    accept and give constructive
        criticism, 123
    accept and give praise, 120
    acknowledge others, 119
    apologize earnestly, 121
    art of caring, 124–125
    assert yourself, 121–122
    avoid personal questions, 122
    be agreeable, 121
    be considerate guest, 122
    be exclusive, 119–120
    cardinal teachings, 125
    care for your guests, 122
    do not speak ill, 120
    don't shift responsibility and
        blame, 123–124
    environment and be gentle,
        animals, 123
    keep it down and rediscover
        silence, 121
    listen, 119
    mind your body, 120
    pay attention, 119
    refrain from idle complaints, 123
    respect even a subtle "no", 120
    respect other people's time and
        space, 121
    respect other's opinions, 120
    speak kindly, 120
    technique illustration, 124
    think the best, 119
    think twice before asking for
        favors, 122

S
Schweitzer, Albert
    AS-1963-343, 69
    AS-1963-526, 69, 70
    AS-GCN-20, 69, 70
    brothers and sisters, suffering, 72
    description, 68–69
    improve social health, 73
    Karsh# 1, 69, 71
    life of compassion and
        service, 72
    living in accordance, 73

    medical missionary, 71
    nursing students, 71
    as physician, philosopher and
        Nobel Prize winner, 69
    The Quest of the Historical
        Jesus, 69
    revelation description, 72
    state-of-the-art, 73
Stuart, Marian R., 129, 131

T
Tardive dyskinesia (TD), 151, 152,
    154
Taylor, Robert B., 140
TD. See Tardive dyskinesia (TD)
Tolstoy's questions, 7
True poetry of life
    American poet, Williams, 140
    healers, 139
    memorable events, authors, 140
    structural violence, 139
Tuo, Hua, 30–31

W
Wagner-Martin, L., 140
Watts, Daniel, 7
Williams, William Carlos, 140
Woodward, Theodore E.
    bioterrorism presentation, 80
    Chairman of Medicine, 77, 78
    class of 1983, 80
    common things occur
        commonly, 79
    researcher, academician and
        trailblazer, 78
    Rickettsial diseases, 77
    sense of humor, 79
    slip doctor, 79
    teaching and commitment, 77
    work ethic and sense of duty, 79
Wooten, Jim, 167

Y
Younger clinicians
    good communication, 112–113

Kalamazoo consensus statement
(*see* Kalamazoo consensus
statement)
practice, 109–112
presentation art (*see* Art of
presentation, younger
clinicians)

Young physician/physician-in-
training, 5

Z
Zhongjing, Zhang, 29–30

CPSIA information can be obtained
at www.ICGtesting.com
Printed in the USA
LVOW10s1501260517
535846LV00022B/136/P